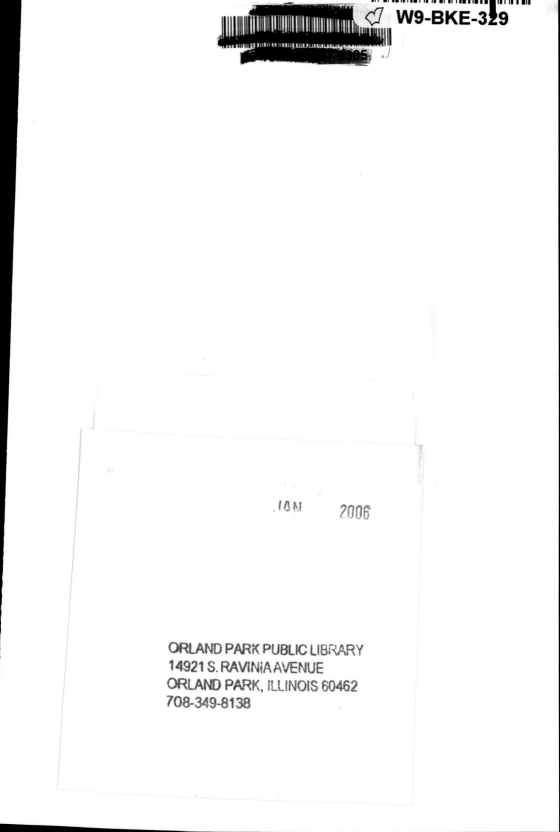

W9-BKE-329

JAN 2006

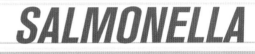

DEADLY DISEASES AND EPIDEMICS

SALMONELLA

Anthrax

Botulism

Campylobacteriosis

Cholera

Ebola

Encephalitis

Escherichia coli Infections

Gonorrhea

Hepatitis

Herpes

HIV/AIDS

Human Papillomavirus and Warts

Influenza

Leprosy

Lyme Disease

Mad Cow Disease (Bovine Spongiform Encephalopathy)

Malaria

Meningitis

Mononucleosis

Pelvic Inflammatory Disease

Plague

Polio

Salmonella

SARS

Smallpox

Streptococcus (Group A)

Staphylococcus aureus Infections

Syphilis

Toxic Shock Syndrome

Tuberculosis

Typhoid Fever

West Nile Virus

DEADLY DISEASES AND EPIDEMICS

SALMONELLA

Danielle A. Brands

FOUNDING EDITOR
The Late **I. Edward Alcamo**
Distinguished Teaching Professor of Microbiology,
SUNY Farmingdale

FOREWORD BY
David Heymann
World Health Organization

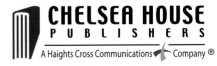

CHELSEA HOUSE
P U B L I S H E R S
A Haights Cross Communications Company ®
Philadelphia

CHELSEA HOUSE PUBLISHERS

VP, NEW PRODUCT DEVELOPMENT Sally Cheney
DIRECTOR OF PRODUCTION Kim Shinners
CREATIVE MANAGER Takeshi Takahashi
MANUFACTURING MANAGER Diann Grasse

Staff for *Salmonella*

EXECUTIVE EDITOR Tara Koellhoffer
ASSOCIATE EDITOR Beth Reger
EDITORIAL ASSISTANT Kuorkor Dzani
PRODUCTION EDITOR Noelle Nardone
PHOTO EDITOR Sarah Bloom
SERIES DESIGNER Terry Mallon
COVER DESIGNER Keith Trego
LAYOUT 21st Century Publishing and Communications, Inc.

Library of Congress Cataloging-in-Publication Data

Brands, Danielle A.
  Salmonella / Danielle A. Brands.
    p. cm.—(Deadly diseases and epidemics)
  Includes bibliographical references.
ISBN 0-7910-8500-7
  1. Salmonellosis. 2. Salmonella. I. Title. II. Series.
RC182.S12B736 2005
615.9'529344—dc22

                                                    2005005348

All links and web addresses were checked and verified to be correct at the time of publication. Because of the dynamic nature of the web, some addresses and links may have changed since publication and may no longer be valid.

Table of Contents

Foreword

In the 1960s, many of the infectious diseases that had terrorized generations were tamed. After a century of advances, the leading killers of Americans both young and old were being prevented with new vaccines or cured with new medicines. The risk of death from pneumonia, tuberculosis (TB), meningitis, influenza, whooping cough, and diphtheria declined dramatically. New vaccines lifted the fear that summer would bring polio, and a global campaign was on the verge of eradicating smallpox worldwide. New pesticides like DDT cleared mosquitoes from homes and fields, thus reducing the incidence of malaria, which was present in the southern United States and which remains a leading killer of children worldwide. New technologies produced safe drinking water and removed the risk of cholera and other water-borne diseases. Science seemed unstoppable. Disease seemed destined to all but disappear.

But the euphoria of the 1960s has evaporated.

The microbes fought back. Those causing diseases like TB and malaria evolved resistance to cheap and effective drugs. The mosquito developed the ability to defuse pesticides. New diseases emerged, including AIDS, Legionnaires, and Lyme disease. And diseases which had not been seen in decades re-emerged, as the hantavirus did in the Navajo Nation in 1993. Technology itself actually created new health risks. The global transportation network, for example, meant that diseases like West Nile virus could spread beyond isolated regions and quickly become global threats. Even modern public health protections sometimes failed, as they did in 1993 in Milwaukee, Wisconsin, resulting in 400,000 cases of the digestive system illness cryptosporidiosis. And, more recently, the threat from smallpox, a disease believed to be completely eradicated, has returned along with other potential bioterrorism weapons such as anthrax.

The lesson is that the fight against infectious diseases will never end.

In our constant struggle against disease, we as individuals have a weapon that does not require vaccines or drugs, and that is the warehouse of knowledge. We learn from the history of science that "modern" beliefs can be wrong. In this series of books, for example, you will learn that diseases like syphilis were once thought to be caused by eating potatoes. The invention of the microscope set science on the right path. There are more positive lessons from history. For example, smallpox was eliminated by vaccinating everyone who had come in contact with an infected person. This "ring" approach to smallpox control is still the preferred method for confronting an outbreak, should the disease be intentionally reintroduced.

At the same time, we are constantly adding new drugs, new vaccines, and new information to the warehouse. Recently, the entire human genome was decoded. So too was the genome of the parasite that causes malaria. Perhaps by looking at the microbe and the victim through the lens of genetics we will be able to discover new ways to fight malaria, which remains the leading killer of children in many countries.

Because of advances in our understanding of such diseases as AIDS, entire new classes of anti-retroviral drugs have been developed. But resistance to all these drugs has already been detected, so we know that AIDS drug development must continue.

Education, experimentation, and the discoveries that grow out of them are the best tools to protect health. Opening this book may put you on the path of discovery. I hope so, because new vaccines, new antibiotics, new technologies, and, most importantly, new scientists are needed now more than ever if we are to remain on the winning side of this struggle against microbes.

David Heymann
Executive Director
Communicable Diseases Section
World Health Organization
Geneva, Switzerland

1

Salmonella Strikes at the Senior Prom

It was finally the Saturday night all four of them had waited for—senior prom night. Mike and Michelle were going with their best friends, Dave and Jodi. Everything was all set: The dresses and tuxedoes were tailored and pressed, and the limousine would arrive at 6:00 P.M. to take them to a fancy restaurant for dinner. After the girls spent the day at the salon getting their hair, makeup, and nails done, it was time to leave. Mike and Dave arrived at Jodi's parents' house to pick up the girls. After posing for several rounds of pictures, they were in the limo and on their way to dinner.

At dinner, everyone was excited as they tried to decide what to eat. Because it was a special occasion, they chose an appetizer of oysters on the half shell. For dinner, Mike and Dave had steaks, and Jodi and Michelle had fish. They were all amazed at how good the food was and decided to order dessert as well. They shared a chocolate mountain cake and a bottle of sparkling cider. Before long, they were all completely stuffed and happy to be back in the limo on their way to the hotel where their prom was being held.

When they arrived, the photographer took their pictures. Soon afterward, they were dancing the night away. The music was great and they were all enjoying the moment. They danced, laughed, and talked until the prom ended at 1:00 A.M. Since they were still too excited to go home and the girls' curfew was not until 2:00 A.M., they decided to drive around for a while and maybe get some coffee.

Once they were back in the limo, Mike realized he was not feeling well. He knew that if he did not get to a bathroom quickly he would have an accident. He was not sure why his stomach was suddenly bothering him. He did not want to make a big deal of the situation in front of the girls. Mike tried to ignore the feeling and hoped it would go away, but it only got worse. Mike had to ask the limo driver to pull over at the next available place, which happened to be an all-night fast-food restaurant. Mike threw open the limo door and dashed into the bathroom, which confused the rest of the group. However, they made the best of the stop by getting ice cream cones. Meanwhile, Mike was having a severe case of diarrhea and was completely embarrassed. He could not believe this was happening to him at a time like this. After about 15 minutes, he was feeling a little better and went outside to join the rest of the group. He was hoping that he would be all right. When he returned, his concerned friends asked if he was okay. Not wanting to tell them what had really happened, he just said he had a stomachache. They decided to call it a night and the limo took everyone home.

Once he got home, Mike had three more bouts of diarrhea and he finally took some Imodium AD® to see if that would stop the episodes. He felt like he had a fever, but he just wanted to rest. Finally, he was able to get to sleep.

At around 6:00 the next morning, Jodi awoke from a deep sleep with severe pains in her stomach. At first, she thought they were menstrual cramps, even though she was not yet due for her period. She took two pain relievers and went back to bed, only to wake up again a few hours later with more stomach cramping and an unusually strong urge to go to the bathroom. Jodi started having watery diarrhea that was tinged with blood. She also had a fever, nausea, and a head-ache. She was very upset that she was getting what she thought was the flu, after having so much fun at the prom the night before. She spent most of the day in bed, and had continuing bouts of diarrhea. Her parents gave her Pepto-Bismol® and plenty of fluids.

Also that morning, Mike was up and about. He was feeling a little better, but his stomach was still queasy and he definitely did not want to eat anything, just in case. His parents made sure he drank water and gave him Tylenol® to bring down his fever.

Meanwhile, Dave and Michelle were feeling just fine and had no idea about what Mike and Jodi were experiencing. Dave had called Jodi on Sunday afternoon to see what she was up to and she said she thought she was coming down with the flu so she was going to hang out at home. Mike had told Michelle that he was fine, just tired, and wanted to stay home and rest.

On Monday, everyone showed up for school and went about their day as usual. Jodi was still not feeling well. She was still getting occasional stomach cramps, but she was just having a few loose stools, not full-blown diarrhea. Mike was feeling fine except for a headache, but he was not worried about it, since he was not having any more diarrhea.

On Wednesday, Mike, Jodi, and Dave were surprised when Michelle failed to show up for school. That was very unlike her; she never missed school. At lunch, they called Michelle to see how she was doing and she just said she was sick with the flu, so they let her go back to sleep. She had a high fever with severe diarrhea and cramping. This continued for three days, and finally, when she started to have bloody diarrhea, she knew she had to go to the doctor. By now, it was Friday, and she called Mike to cancel her plans with him, Dave, and Jodi that night. Mike told her that Dave was sick, too.

That afternoon, Michelle told her doctor about her symptoms and how long she had had them. The doctor took a stool sample for testing to see what was wrong. The doctor told her to get plenty of fluids and rest. He said he would call the next day with her test results.

The next morning, the doctor called and said that Michelle had **salmonellosis**, a form of food poisoning. He asked her what she had eaten over the past few days and whether anyone who had eaten the same foods was sick, but she could not think of anything. The doctor prescribed an **antibiotic** called ciprofloxacin. He told Michelle to take the medication for five days with plenty of fluids. He told her that she should be feeling better in about three days.

On Saturday afternoon, Michelle called Jodi and explained the whole situation. Jodi wondered if she had had the same problem the day after the prom. Jodi called Dave and they talked about what Michelle's doctor had told her and they wondered if that was what they had had, too. Dave was still sick, though he was having only a few bouts of occasional diarrhea, so he decided to go to his doctor.

On Sunday, Dave found out that he, too, had salmonellosis. The four friends tried to figure out if that was what all of them had. They all felt stupid for hiding the fact that they had been sick from each other; if they had been honest, they might have found out sooner what was wrong. They decided to look on the Internet and read about salmonellosis and *Salmonella*, the **bacterium** that causes the disease. They were amazed that it was possible to come down with salmonellosis anywhere from six hours to four days after eating contaminated food. They tried to recall what they had eaten that might have made them sick. Realizing that the only meal they had in common was the dinner on the night of their prom, they thought about what they had eaten. Jodi remembered that the only thing they all ate were the oysters and cake. They looked on the Internet and discovered that oysters are a common source of *Salmonella* (Figure 1.1). They decided that this was probably what had caused their illness. They also decided then and there that they would never eat oysters again!

Cases of food poisoning, such as salmonellosis, often go misdiagnosed or undiagnosed. Most people just assume they

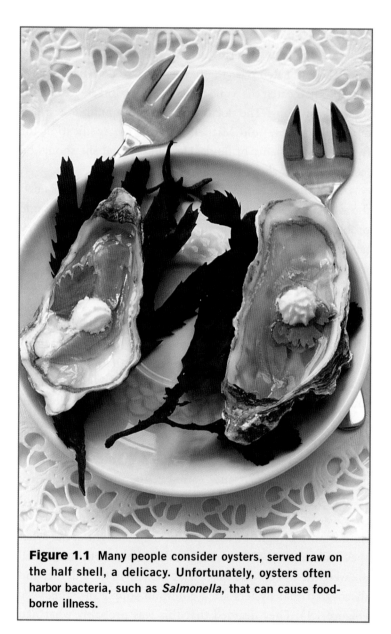

Figure 1.1 Many people consider oysters, served raw on the half shell, a delicacy. Unfortunately, oysters often harbor bacteria, such as *Salmonella*, that can cause food-borne illness.

have the flu and do not get proper treatment for the problem. Often, cases go completely unnoticed. When you get salmonellosis, you may not get a severe infection. You may just get a

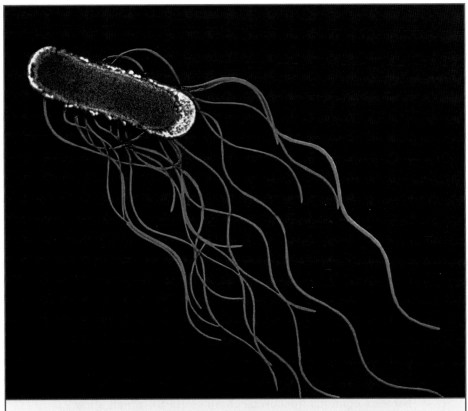

Figure 1.2 Shown here is a transmission electron micrograph (TEM) of a single *Salmonella* bacterium, magnified 13,250 times. The long stringy structures protruding from the bacterium are called flagella, which the bacterium uses to move.

headache and a mild stomachache. This makes documenting cases of **food-borne illness** a challenge for doctors.

This book will examine the *Salmonella* bacterium (Figure 1.2), investigate salmonellosis, and discuss why there has been an increase in salmonellosis cases, possible sources for infection with *Salmonella*, how it makes you sick, and how your body reacts to this bacterium. We will also examine the role that animals play in human cases of salmonellosis, how to treat infections, and how to prevent infections.

SALMONELLA THE BACTERIUM

Salmonella is a type of **organism** called a bacterium (the plural is *bacteria*). More specifically, *Salmonella* is a type of bacterium called a **bacillus**, a name given to all bacteria that have the rod-like shape seen in Figure 1.3. Scientists use other terms to classify *Salmonella* and other bacteria that share certain characteristics. These terms include **gram-negative**, which describes bacteria (including *Salmonella*) that have a thick double cell wall that causes them to lose a violet stain when

GRAM-NEGATIVE AND GRAM-POSITIVE BACTERIA

The Gram stain technique, invented in 1844 by Hans Christian Gram, helps classify bacteria, dividing them into two groups: gram-positive and gram-negative. The difference between the two groups is in the cell wall of the bacterium. Gram-positive bacteria have cell walls that contain many layers of peptidoglycan, which consists of sugars and peptide chains that form a thick rigid structure. Gram-negative bacteria have very few layers of peptidoglycan. The outer membrane of gram-negative bacteria contains lipopolysaccharides (LPS), which allow the immune system to destroy the bacteria. Gram-negative bacteria have such a small amount of peptidoglycan that the cell breaks easily.

To perform a Gram stain test, cells are first "fixed" to a slide by passing the slide quickly through a flame. The cells are then stained with crystal violet dye, and then rinsed. A second stain, called a counterstain, is then applied to the slide and rinsed. Cells that keep the initial crystal violet stain appear purple when examined under a microscope, and are considered gram-positive. Cells that do not hold onto this initial stain instead pick up the color of the counterstain and appear pink or red. These cells are considered gram-negative.

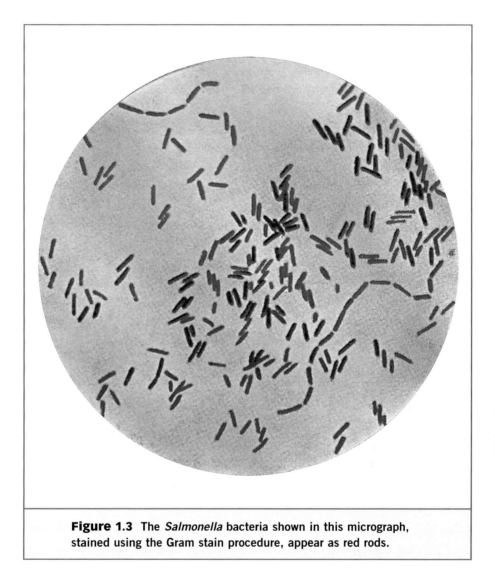

Figure 1.3 The *Salmonella* bacteria shown in this micrograph, stained using the Gram stain procedure, appear as red rods.

rinsed during certain laboratory tests, and **anaerobic**, which means "capable of living and growing without oxygen." (*Salmonella* does not need oxygen to survive, but it does prefer to grow in an oxygen-rich environment.) Like many other kinds of bacteria, *Salmonella* is able to produce **infection** when it enters a person's body.

THE HISTORY OF *SALMONELLA*

Salmonella was first identified in 1885. It was named for one of the two men who discovered it, Daniel Elmer Salmon (the other was Theobald Smith). They first found *Salmonella* in hogs that were ill with a disease called hog cholera. At the time, they named the organism "Hog-cholerabacillus." Today, we call this same organism *Salmonella cholera-suis*. It did not get the name *Salmonella* until the year 1900, when French scientist Joseph Léon Ligniéres suggested calling the entire swine group *Salmonella* in honor of Salmon.

Salmonella was known by many other names before its official title was chosen. It had been called TPE, or typhoid-parathyphus-enteritis. A German bacteriologist named Karl Joseph Eberth referred to it as *Eberthella typhi*. Since its discovery in the late 1800s and its naming in 1900, many additional forms of bacteria have been added to the *Salmonella* group, which now includes more than 2,500 types that are able to infect humans and animals.

TYPES OF *SALMONELLA*

Many different types of *Salmonella* exist, some of which cause illness in both animals and people. Some types cause illness in animals but not in people. The various forms of *Salmonella* that can infect people are referred to as **serotypes**, which are very closely related microorganisms that share certain structural features. Some serotypes are only present in certain parts of the world.

THE STRUCTURE AND FUNCTION OF *SALMONELLA*

Because *Salmonella* is very easy to grow in a laboratory, quite a bit is known about its structure and activity. *Salmonella* is a gram-negative rod that has a growth rate, or division rate, of 40 minutes. *Salmonella* prefers to grow at 37°C (98.6°F), but has the ability to grow at a wide range of temperatures, from 6 to 46°C (43 to 115°F). This provides *Salmonella* with many opportunities to grow.

Luckily for us, *Salmonella* needs more than the proper temperature to grow, it also needs a pH range of 4.1–9.0, which is mildly basic to strongly acidic. Optimum growth occurs at a pH of 6.5–7.5, which is close to neutral, meaning not basic or acidic.

Salmonella also has nutritional requirements that must be met for it to grow and divide. For example, *Salmonella* needs glucose (a sugar) that is very readily available in the human body. In the laboratory, there are usually three main nutrients that are part of the medium in which *Salmonella* is typically grown: yeast (such as the substance used to make bread rise) extract, which is highly nutritious; tryptone, which is a protein found in milk; and sodium chloride (NaCl), also known as table salt. *Salmonella* does not need oxygen to grow; but prefers it. Although it will grow without the presence of oxygen, it may grow at a slower rate.

If all of these factors—proper temperature, pH, and nutrition—are met, *Salmonella* will grow very easily. If you think about it, all of these factors are present in your body, which makes a human body a good **host** for *Salmonella*.

2

Salmonella and Food-borne Illness

Salmonella is responsible for more than 40,000 cases of food-borne illness every year. The incidence of *Salmonella* infections has risen dramatically since the 1980s, leading to high medical costs, a loss of wages for workers who become ill, and a loss of productivity for the companies whose workers do become ill. In all, these financial losses can cost more than $3.6 billion each year.

Salmonella infections have long been a concern to scientists, doctors, and the U.S. Food and Drug Administration (FDA). During the late 1960s, there were numerous outbreaks around the nation of typhoid fever (another disease caused by *Salmonella* infection), which can be food-borne or passed from person to person through poor hygiene practices. Symptoms of typhoid fever include diarrhea and **sepsis**, a toxic condition caused by the spread of bacteria or their products in the bloodstream. Because seafood was a major source of the bacteria that causes typhoid, the FDA put guidelines in place for seafood producers—regulating how long fishermen could be out to sea while there was seafood on the boat, to prevent spoilage. All seafood had to be kept on ice and had to be sent to a distributor within hours of being caught. The FDA also required that waters used for harvesting and fishing be tested for fecal pathogens— disease-causing microorganisms that are found in solid human waste. These regulations led to a significant decrease in the yearly number of cases of typhoid fever.

In the late 1980s, however, infections with new types of *Salmonella* occurred. These infections have become more and more common with each passing year, to the point where they have reached epidemic proportions (an epidemic is a disease outbreak that affects a large number of people within a population, community, or region at the same time). People who get *Salmonella* infections usually develop **gastroenteritis** (inflammation of the stomach and intestines that can cause diarrhea, vomiting, and cramps) but not **enteric fever** (an infection that produces fever, weakness, and inflammation and ulceration of the intestines), which is seen with typhoid fever.

WHAT IS FOOD POISONING?

A person gets food poisoning by eating food or drinking a beverage that contains a disease-causing agent. These agents can be **pathogens** or **chemicals**. When a person consumes a food or beverage that contains one or more of these agents, the agents travel to the stomach and intestines. Once there, they interfere with the body's functions, making the person ill. To date, more than 250 different organisms have been identified that can cause food poisoning. These organisms are grouped into three main categories: bacteria, **viruses**, and **parasites**. As we know from Chapter 1, *Salmonella* is a bacterium.

Food-borne disease is a major problem in the United States, both in the number of yearly cases and in the resulting economic costs. There are approximately 76 million cases of food-borne illness per year, with 325,000 of these cases requiring hospitalization and 5,000 resulting in death.

TWO MISCONCEPTIONS
ABOUT FOOD-BORNE ILLNESS

One of the biggest misconceptions about food poisoning is that it is always caused by the last meal the sick person ate. This is not necessarily true. Although Mike and Jodi showed symptoms soon after eating the oysters on prom night, Dave and Michelle did not become ill until several days later. When someone gets ill, he or she usually only thinks about what he or she ate at the most recent meal. In fact, most food-borne pathogens need a minimum of 12 hours—and sometimes up to 72 hours—to cause disease. The symptoms take a while to develop because once the bacteria pass through the stomach and take hold in the intestine, they still need to multiply and trigger the infected person's **immune response** (the body's reaction to substances that it sees as foreign).

The second misconception about food-borne disease is that the number of annual reported cases is accurate, which may lead public health officials to underestimate how big a problem these diseases really are. The numbers are not a true representation of how common food poisoning is, however, because few people go to the doctor for a case of diarrhea. Instead, most just take over-the-counter medicines (like the Pepto-Bismol Jodi's parents gave her) to try to control the symptoms, and tell as few people about their condition as possible. There is nothing pleasant about constantly running to the bathroom due to attacks of diarrhea—it is perhaps even *less* desirable to hear someone else talk about it. As a result,

THE NATIONAL *SALMONELLA* SURVEILLANCE SYSTEM

The National *Salmonella* Surveillance System has been tracking *Salmonella* **isolates** by serotype since 1968. The Centers for Disease Control and Prevention (CDC) collects isolates of *Salmonella* from humans from all over the United States. These data are reported using the Public Health Laboratory Information System (PHLIS), which connects all of the state health labs together to track the outbreaks, patterns, and geographical distribution of salmonellosis. By pooling all of this information together, scientists are able to track outbreaks, determine where and when they happen, and try to localize where the outbreak first occurred. This system also allows experts to compile statistics on where certain strains are occurring and how prevalent a particular strain is.

there are thousands of unreported cases of food-borne disease every year, which makes it hard for scientists to determine how prevalent food-borne pathogens really are. If individual cases were reported more regularly, outbreaks would be easier to detect and, possibly, easier to prevent.

HOW IS SALMONELLOSIS DETECTED IN A PERSON?

To isolate *Salmonella* from a person, a doctor takes a sample of the person's feces and streaks it on a media plate that contains the nutrients (mentioned earlier) that allow *Salmonella* to grow. The doctor then checks the plate after 24 hours to see if any *Salmonella* colonies are growing (Figure 2.1). A single colony (which can contain 100,000 bacteria), is placed on a slide and viewed under a microscope to look for the common rod shape that is characteristic of *Salmonella*. The doctor can then confirm that the person is suffering from salmonellosis and can begin the appropriate course of treatment.

SYMPTOMS AND COMPLICATIONS OF *SALMONELLA* INFECTIONS

As we saw with the teens in Chapter 1, salmonellosis produces several symptoms. These include diarrhea that may be bloody, stomach cramping that may be severe, fever, and, occasionally, nausea. The onset of symptoms can take anywhere from 6 to 72 hours, but usually occurs around 12 hours after consuming the contaminated food or beverage. As with all other infections, the symptoms vary from person to person, and depend greatly on the patient's current state of health. A person who is **immunocompromised** (has a weakened immune system) may experience a more severe case of food poisoning because the body is unable to fight off the disease as easily as a healthier person's body could. (Certain categories of people are more likely than others to be immunocompromised. These include babies, elderly people, or people who have particular diseases—for example, acquired immunodeficiency syndrome

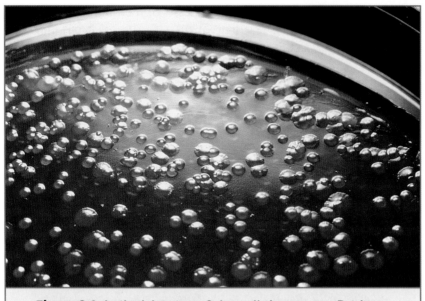

Figure 2.1 In the laboratory, *Salmonella* is grown on Petri dishes as seen here. The Petri dishes contain media that is a nutrient source for the bacteria to grow on. The small round raised surfaces are referred to as colonies. Each colony contains thousands of bacteria.

[AIDS].) In the case of an immunocompromised person, doctors would administer antibiotic treatment quickly—if, that is, the person visits a doctor.

It is estimated that there are more than 500 fatalities a year from salmonellosis. There are several reasons why this disease kills so many people. If a person has severe symptoms but does not go to the doctor, he or she may allow the bacteria to damage the body. Not seeking treatment allows **opportunistic pathogens**—microorganisms that normally live on certain areas of the body without causing harm but can cause disease when they gain access to other areas of the body—to take hold in the body, which forces the body to fight multiple infections at the same time. This often happens in developing countries. Another condition that could cause someone to die from salmonellosis is dehydration. When you have diarrhea, it is extremely important to take in enough fluids. A person has to take in more fluids than he or she excretes. If a person also has a fever, which is often the case with salmonellosis, the need for fluids is even greater. This is because fever elevates body temperature and naturally requires more fluids to help fight the infection and bring the body temperature back down to normal, about 98.6°F (37°C). It is very common for people who have diarrhea to stop drinking fluids, mistakenly believing that if they stop drinking, there will be no liquid to come back out. However, by the time a person feels thirsty, the body is already

APHIS: ANIMAL AND PLANT HEALTH INSPECTION SERVICES

APHIS, the Animal and Plant Health Inspection Services, is a division of the U.S. Department of Agriculture (USDA). APHIS offers a wide range of services. For instance, you can log onto the APHIS Website, *www.aphis.usda.gov*, to find travel information, which includes any restrictions on food or animals at the place you plan to visit. This will provide you with up-to-date information on whether you can bring pets or other animals into Canada, for example. It will also tell you whether you are allowed to bring food, such as exotic fruits, into the United States.

APHIS has the largest laboratory in the United States that identifies different types of *Salmonella*. When someone, such as a farmer, researcher, or environmental agency official, believes he or she has *Salmonella*, that person sends a sample (stool, crop, or media plate) to APHIS. APHIS tests the sample to determine whether it does, in fact, contain *Salmonella*, and if so, which type of *Salmonella*. If there are many samples of one type of *Salmonella* that come from the same area, APHIS is able to determine if there is an outbreak and can help locate the source.

dehydrated. This is true not just with cases of food poisoning; it is a fact for everyday life.

Salmonellosis can cause long-term complications, although this happens in fewer than 2% of cases. The most common long-term problem is a condition called Reiter's syndrome, also known as septic arthritis or **pyogenic** arthritis. It is a serious infection that causes inflammation and swelling in the joints, along with fever, severe pain, chills, and loss of function in the infected joints. It occurs when *Salmonella* bacteria enter the bloodstream and take hold in the joints. Reiter's syndrome can cause severe damage to the bone and cartilage. It is a very painful and serious condition that needs to be treated immediately. Once the bacteria have reached the joints through the bloodstream, it is very easy for the infection to become **systemic**, meaning that the whole body is infected. This is often fatal. Treatment for Reiter's syndrome, if caught early enough, usually consists of a continuous six-week course of antibiotics administered intravenously (IV), through a needle placed into one of the sick person's veins. The pain usually subsides within a few weeks, but it can last for several months. Sometimes joints can be damaged beyond repair, which can cause long-term suffering. In some cases, depending on the extent of the damage, surgery can be performed to replace lost or damaged cartilage. Surgery cannot take place until the patient is completely free from infection, however; otherwise, there would be a risk of spreading the bacteria to other parts of the body during the operation.

HOW MANY BACTERIA DOES IT TAKE TO MAKE YOU SICK?

Salmonella has the ability to cause infection with only a small amount of bacteria present. This is one of the reasons why there are so many cases of salmonellosis each year. To cause an infection, at least 300 bacteria must be present in the body. This is a relatively small amount, compared with the 1,000 to 20,000 organisms that are needed to cause many other diseases. If there are 300 *Salmonella* bacteria present on your chicken sandwich, it does not necessarily mean you will get sick, however. Your body has some natural defenses to protect you. You will only get sick if the bacteria take hold in your intestines and are able to outcompete the **normal flora** (the bacteria that live naturally in your gut).

Like other parts of the body, the intestines provide a home for some forms of bacteria. These bacteria do not harm the body, and, in some cases, they are actually helpful—for

THE BACTERIA THAT LIVE IN YOUR GUT

Normal flora will not make you sick, but you may notice them when you travel to a new place or country. You may get intestinal upset, also known as traveler's diarrhea. This comes from eating foods and drinking water that are different from what you normally consume. New foods and beverages may contain types of bacteria that are different from those that make up your normal flora. Some countries also have poor waste treatment facilities, which allow pathogens to enter drinking water. People from developed countries—where the water is cleaner—may be more prone to disease because their immune systems are not used to fighting some of these pathogens.

You may also become ill when you take antibiotics for an infection, such as strep throat, and might suffer from diarrhea after the first few days of taking the medication. This is because antibiotics can wipe out your normal flora. The antibiotic does not know that it is only supposed to kill the bacteria that cause the strep throat; instead, it kills all bacteria that it can. The diarrhea comes from the body's attempt to reestablish its normal flora as you eat. In this case, some bacteria that would not normally make you sick will cause diarrhea until your intestinal tract's normal flora have returned.

example, some types of bacteria aid in digestion. The normal flora do not cause a person to get sick, but they are always present. They establish themselves in the gut shortly after birth from organisms that are present in the **colostrum** in breast milk, cow's milk, and the first foods a child eats. They are constantly regenerated or replaced through the foods we eat.

When *Salmonella* bacteria come into contact with the intestines, they first have to find a **niche** to colonize. Once they have found a niche, the bacteria must then multiply to out-number the normal bacterial population before they can cause infection. Once the infectious level is reached, the victim will experience the symptoms of disease. This process of infection is the same whether the bacteria are trying to infect a person or an animal. In Chapter 3, we will take a closer look at the relationship between *Salmonella*, the animals it infects, and how infections in animals relate to infections in people.

3

Hosts, Sources, and Carriers

People are not the only living organisms that get salmonellosis. Many other kinds of animals also come down with the illness. When animals get the disease, they show the same symptoms that people do.

Animals play a huge role in human cases of salmonellosis. Foods produced from animals that have been raised on a farm, caught by fishermen, or harvested through **aquaculture** (the farming of plants and animals that live in water) are the leading sources of *Salmonella* infections in people. Between the farm or aquaculture facility, butchering process, and dinner preparation, there are ample opportunities for animal carcasses to become contaminated with *Salmonella*. Once contaminated food gets into people's homes, if the food is not handled properly, it is easy for anyone or anything that eats the food to become infected.

Salmonellosis is particularly costly to ranchers. If an animal loses too much weight due to illness, there will not be enough meat to sell for profit. In addition, the cost of treating infections is high. For these reasons alone, ranchers frequently use feeds that have been supplemented with antibiotics to prevent salmonellosis and other bacterial infections in their animals. Some consumers refuse to buy and eat products that came from food animals that have been given feeds containing antibiotics, which increases the financial costs to the rancher by reducing the number of people who will buy the rancher's products.

Besides sheep, goats, cattle, chickens, and pigs, some of the other animals that can become infected with *Salmonella* include geese and other birds, lizards and other reptiles, shellfish, and amphibians such as turtles. Animals can actually pass *Salmonella* on to other animals, as well as to people. A disease that can be transferred from animals to people is known as a **zoonosis** (the plural is *zoonoses*).

ANIMALS AS CARRIERS AND SOURCES OF *SALMONELLA*

Both animals and people can be **reservoirs** for *Salmonella*. That is, they can carry the bacteria and not suffer from an active infection. In this situation, the bacteria stay in the intestines as part of the living thing's normal flora. It is quite common for "carriers" to exist for a disease. This means that a person can transmit the disease, such as salmonellosis, to others without the carrier actually being sick. You will see a famous example of this later in this chapter when you read the story of Typhoid Mary. Some insects, such as mosquitoes, are also carriers. Mosquitoes can harbor diseases such as West Nile virus, and they can transmit the disease to a human through their bite. Whenever the animal **defecates** (has a bowel movement), it **sheds** (releases pathogens from the body into the environment) the bacteria in its feces. All of this can happen without the particular animal ever actually getting sick. Animals defecating and shedding the bacteria into the environment and the bacteria then entering the food supply—for example, on crops—is a common method of human *Salmonella* contamination.

Cattle and chicken are the two main animal sources of human *Salmonella* infections. When animals are prepared for slaughter and processing, they are handled by many different workers. If *Salmonella* or any other pathogen is present on the equipment or on the workers' hands or clothing, contamination is possible. Most often, contamination occurs during certain stages of slaughter: bleeding, skinning (or feather removal for chickens), **evisceration** (removal of the contents of the chest and belly, also known as gutting), and the handling of carcasses prior to processing.

Besides cattle and poultry (chicken, turkey, duck, and pheasants), other food products can be a source of *Salmonella*. Shellfish, for instance, are a major cause of salmonellosis in people—as the teens in Chapter 1 learned the hard way. Oysters, clams, and mussels are **filter feeders**. This means that they get their food out of the water that flows through their bodies. In the process, they also ingest anything else that happens to be in the water. Oceans, lakes, and bays are heavily contaminated with fecal matter. Also, animals that live near streams and lakes defecate in the water, which then flows into the bays and oceans from which shellfish are harvested. The shellfish take in any pathogens present in the water and then hold them in their intestines. The biggest problem is with oysters, since they are most often eaten raw on the half shell. There may be enough bacteria present in a single raw oyster to cause an infection in the human gut. Mussels and clams, on the other hand, pose less of a risk because they are usually steamed and thorough cooking kills *Salmonella* bacteria.

These are only a few of the ways that animals and animal products cause *Salmonella* infection. It is a problem of such importance, however, that food animal producers and public health regulators continue to debate possible strategies for reducing contamination in the nation's food supply.

OTHER FOODS THAT CAN CARRY *SALMONELLA*

Cattle, chicken, and shellfish are not the only food animals that can cause a person to become infected with *Salmonella*. Other animals that can harbor *Salmonella* include turkeys, sheep, and swine.

Some nonanimal food products can also carry *Salmonella* bacteria. Fruits and vegetables such as cantaloupes, melons, tomatoes, lettuce, and especially alfalfa sprouts have been linked to cases of salmonellosis in humans. There are several different routes through which these products can become contaminated. The water used to irrigate crops can be contaminated with animal fecal matter. Also, the manure used as fertilizer—which is made from cow feces—may contain *Salmonella* if the animal was shedding the bacteria when the fertilizer was produced. Some farmworkers—for example, day laborers who are hired to help out during harvest time—may not follow the strict health regulations observed by professional farmers. The workers may use the fields as bathrooms, urinating and defecating near or even on the crops that end up in your kitchen.

Some ways to reduce the risk of illness from fruits and vegetable is to wash all fresh foods thoroughly. Unfortunately, this precaution does not work for alfalfa sprouts and lettuce. When these vegetables are washed, the bacteria are forced deeper into the lower layers of lettuce leaves or sprouts. The best way to handle these foods is to peel off the outside three layers of lettuce, where the contamination would be, and then

SALMONELLA AND MARIJUANA

One other source that can contain *Salmonella* that most people would never think about is marijuana. Hopefully, you already know how dangerous it is to use marijuana, but in case you might consider it, here are some facts you should know. Marijuana leaves harbor *Salmonella* very readily. In fact, just touching the leaves may lead to an infection with *Salmonella*. As with any plant or crop, the water used to grow marijuana is not necessarily clean. Also, the people who deal with this illegal substance are not often concerned about handling it safely. You probably already know that you should stay away from marijuana, but now you can also consider whether it is worth the risk of dying from an infection with *Salmonella*.

eat only the inside layers. Sprouts need to be separated and then washed carefully.

Many of the other foods that can carry *Salmonella* are items that people might not normally consider a source of contamination. Just about everyone has heard warnings about the need to handle raw chicken properly and to cook chicken and eggs thoroughly to avoid *Salmonella* contamination. But who has ever heard warnings about the handling or preparation of almonds, pecans, or chocolate? These foods are also possible sources of *Salmonella*.

OTHER SOURCES OF INFECTION FOR *SALMONELLA*

Some sources of *Salmonella* include kitchen countertops

"SUSPECT ALMONDS FORCE RECALL OF GRANOLA, MUESLI."

Almonds from Paramount Farms of California were recalled because they were contaminated with *Salmonella*. Granola bars with expiration dates between June 6, 2004 and January 20, 2005 were recalled. The granola bars were mostly store brand granola bars, and fruit and trail mix, sold under the names Acme®, Albertsons®, BI-LO®, Food Club®, Food Lion®, Fred Meyer®, Giant®, Giant Eagle®, Great Value®, Hill Country Fare®, Hyvee®, Jewel®, Kroger®, Laura Lynn®, Meijer®, Millville®, Our Family®, Price Chopper®, Ralph's®, Roundy®, Stater Brothers®, Stop & Shop®, Sunny Select®, Tops®, Weis®, and Winn Dixie®. Muesli was also recalled with the expiration dates of September 10, 2004 and December 10, 2004. The stores that sold this product are: Acme, Albertsons, Archer Farm®, Best Choice®, Central Market®, Flavorite®, Fred Meyer®, Harris Teeter®, Hyvee, Jewel, Kroger, Ralph's, Safeway Select Healthy Advantage®, Shaws®, and Shop 'N Save®.

Arizona Daily Star, Thursday, July 15, 2004, Section A5, Associated Press, Washington.

where contaminated food has been placed. Other possible sources are doorknobs and toilets that infected people have recently touched, although the bacteria cannot survive long on these types of surfaces. Objects such doorknobs or countertops are called **fomites**—inanimate objects that can spread germs (pathogens) and cause disease. For example, if a classmate sneezes on a computer mouse or keyboard and then you use it, you will have the other person's germs on your hands. The germs that are now on your hands can go inside your body if you touch your mouth or other mucous membranes. This form of pathogen transmission is very common in day-care centers, since babies and toddlers drool on the toys and share them, and rarely wash their hands. Pets can also pass *Salmonella* to their owners. Pets frequently sniff fecal matter outside and may step in feces and then track it into the home.

Environmental sources of *Salmonella* include water, soil, and insects. Water and soil that contain fecal matter, or are touched by flies that have landed on fecal matter, can easily come into contact with food products. Water is a hazard in states that allow recycled wastewater to be used to water yards and crops. This practice spreads contaminants from the recycled wastewater to the lawn on which your family and pets play and to the garden from which your family gets its fresh vegetables (Figure 3.1).

TYPHOID FEVER

Typhoid fever is a dreaded, often deadly disease caused by a form of *Salmonella* called *Salmonella typhi*. The bacterium that causes typhoid was first identified in the 1880s. Water is the main route through which this pathogen is transmitted.

Typhoid fever is characterized by a high, extended fever and diarrhea. Before antibiotics came into widespread use in the 1940s, the **fatality rate** (the number of deaths that occur in a population over a given amount of time) from typhoid was

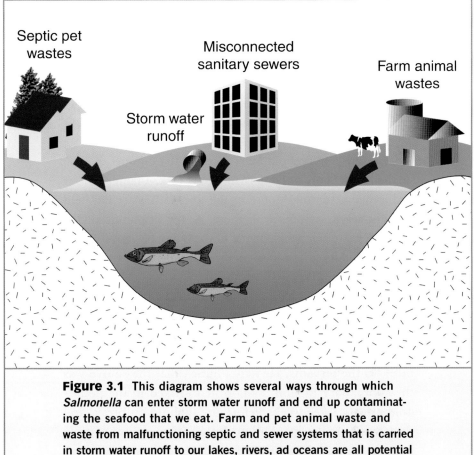

Septic pet wastes

Misconnected sanitary sewers

Farm animal wastes

Storm water runoff

Figure 3.1 This diagram shows several ways through which *Salmonella* can enter storm water runoff and end up contaminating the seafood that we eat. Farm and pet animal waste and waste from malfunctioning septic and sewer systems that is carried in storm water runoff to our lakes, rivers, ad oceans are all potential sources for *Salmonella* contamination. Fish living in these contaminated waters become infected by *Salmonella* and, in turn, pass along the bacteria when they are consumed for food.

about 20%. Since antibiotics were discovered, the fatality rate has decreased significantly. The bacterium that causes typhoid is not one of the more common forms of *Salmonella* today, thanks to government regulations put into place in the 1980s that placed strict guidelines on water treatment. In the early years of the 20th century, however, the pathogen that caused typhoid fever was common and extremely dangerous.

Typhoid Mary: A Famous
Case of *Salmonella*'s Spread

As you will recall, animals—and sometimes people—are reservoirs of *Salmonella*, capable of having the bacteria inside their bodies and spreading it to others, even if they never become ill themselves. One of the most famous examples of this phenomenon involved a woman known to history as "Typhoid Mary."

The story of Typhoid Mary starts in the summer of 1906 on the North Shore of Long Island, New York. A family of four had rented a summer house in the town of Oyster Bay, and brought seven servants with them. At the beginning of the summer, six of the people living in the house became infected with typhoid fever. The local public health department investigated the house to try to determine the source of the outbreak, but could not find the cause. The situation worried the owner of the house, so he hired George Soper, a sanitation engineer, to try to figure out what was causing the illness.

Soper was able to narrow down the cause of the outbreak to the servants. He had a hunch that the source was the cook, Mary Mallon. Mallon had arrived in the household exactly three weeks before the typhoid outbreak, and three weeks is the **incubation period** (the amount of time between a person's exposure to a disease-causing agent and the first appearance of symptoms) for typhoid fever. Soper could not ignore the coincidence of the cook's arrival at the house and the time when the residents fell ill. To confirm his theory, he looked into some of the foods that Mallon had cooked for the family and found that she had made a dessert of ice cream mixed with fresh peaches. Soper knew that fruit and dairy products can easily transmit pathogens. Because handwashing was not a common practice at the time, Soper surmised that Mallon was transmitting the bacteria, which were shed in her feces, to the foods she prepared and served to her employers.

To confirm that he was correct about Mallon, Soper contacted the New York agency through which the family had hired her. He investigated her previous cooking jobs. As he expected, he found that typhoid fever had broken out among nearly all of her previous employers who ate the food she had prepared. By the time Soper determined this, Mallon had already moved on to a new cooking job for a family living in a house on Park Avenue in New York City. When he arrived, there were already two cases of typhoid fever, one of them a little girl who had died from the illness. Soper now knew that he had found the typhoid carrier.

Hoping to put a stop to the outbreaks that Mallon was causing, Soper went to talk to her, hoping to enlist her help. Much to his dismay, she refused to acknowledge the problem. Mary Mallon was about 40 years old. She was educated, well read, and knew how to write well. More than anything, Mallon loved to cook. It was her way of life. So, when Soper approached her with his theories, she refused to listen to him. He wondered if she did not already suspect that something was wrong, since wherever she went, typhoid outbreaks occurred and she never worked for the same family for very long. Soper asked her if she would submit samples of her feces for testing to determine whether she was a carrier of the *Salmonella* bacterium that causes typhoid fever. Her reaction was to grab a carving fork from the table and chase him out of the house.

Realizing he was not going to get any help from Mallon, Soper reported her to the board of health. The board of health sent regulatory officials, an ambulance, interns, and Dr. S. Josephine Baker in response to Soper's request. When they arrived at the house and knocked on the door of the servants' entrance, Mallon answered and quickly understood what they wanted. Mallon fled from the house. The board of health personnel were unable to find her until a policeman found footprints in the snow leading away from the house and toward a neighbor's home. They searched the neighbor's house for three hours before Mallon was found hiding in a closet. When the police found her, she had to be carried kicking and screaming to the hospital.

At the hospital, tests determined that Mallon was indeed carrying *Salmonella typhi*. Baker and Soper tried to reason with Mallon, but she just looked at them angrily. They explained that she could be released if she promised never to work as a cook again and to check in regularly with the health department. Mallon refused their offers, unable to believe that she could be spreading the disease if she was not sick herself. Mallon was moved to Riverside Hospital, located on an island in the East River, and was held there for three years. During her detention in the hospital, the media publicized her case and dubbed her "Typhoid Mary." Eventually, she agreed to stay in touch with the health department and not to cook professionally, so the hospital released her. For a while, she earned a living by washing clothes, but she soon vanished and the authorities could not track her down.

Mallon knew that she would not be able to work as a cook in private homes, so she took jobs instead in several hotels and institutions. Just as had happened before with the families she cooked for, typhoid fever broke out in the hotels and institutions where she was employed. To avoid getting caught by the authorities, she moved quickly from job to job. Health officials finally found her in 1915. At that time, she was working at the Sloane Maternity Hospital in Manhattan, New York, where a large typhoid outbreak occurred. At least 25 hospital employees came down with the illness, and 2 of them died. Mallon was identified and captured. This time, she went quietly.

"Typhoid Mary" was sent back to Riverside Hospital on North Brother Island. She spent the remaining 23 years of her life there, before dying of pneumonia in 1938. In all, some 47 cases of typhoid—three of them fatal—had been linked to her (Figure 3.2).

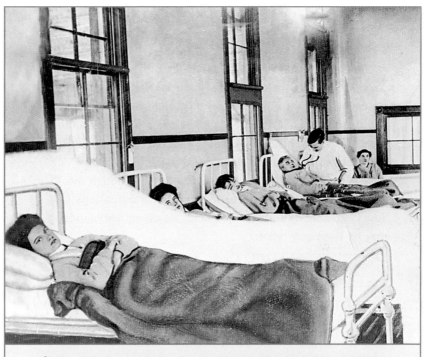

Figure 3.2 Seen here in a hospital bed in New York (at front) is the woman dubbed Typhoid Mary. She was quarantined after infecting many individuals through her work as a cook. She was the first reported carrier of the Salmonella bacteria that cause typhoid.

Mallon's case showed how dangerous "healthy carriers" could be. Eventually, a better understanding of how good hygiene can prevent the spread of pathogens helped make people aware that they should handle food with care. This increased awareness has helped greatly decrease dangerous *Salmonella* outbreaks like the one associated with "Typhoid Mary."

As you can see from this chapter, people as well as animals can be carriers of disease. **Asymptomatic** carriers, who may not even know they carry an infection, can continually pass the bacteria on to unsuspecting hosts. For example, when you have a cold, you cover your mouth when you sneeze and cough to avoid passing the infection to others. Another way carriers may

STOMACH ACID, BACTERIA, AND ULCERS

Helicobacter pylori is one of the types of bacteria that, like *Salmonella*, can survive in the acidic environment of the stomach. This is a very common bacterium that you often hear about in drug advertisements on television. The common name for the condition caused by *Helicobacter pylori* is an ulcer. Some ulcers are caused by this bacterium, in which case they can be treated with antibiotics. Although most people can simply take over-the-counter medications like Tums® to combat the stomach acid, for others antibiotics may be their only relief.

spread illness is the **fecal-oral route**, which is the way Mary Mallon was able to transfer the bacteria to the people who ate the food she prepared. She did not wash her hands properly after using the restroom before she handled food. If you are not even aware that you are contagious, you can infect a large number of people, which is why having good hygiene is important, as you will see in Chapter 8.

4

Salmonella in the Body

The human stomach is filled with juices that are very acidic. The acids in these juices help the stomach break down food so that the nutrients can be used by the body. You might wonder why the stomach acid does not kill *Salmonella* when it invades the body. The fact is that some bacteria actually like to live in acidic conditions. *Salmonella* bacteria have the ability to grow in acidic environments, as you read in Chapter 2.

The level of acid in the stomach is not constant. The amount of food present in the stomach is one factor that changes the amount of acid present. For instance, if a person eats a big meal of steak, a baked potato, and vegetables, then washes it down with a glass of milk, the acid in the stomach is put to work breaking down the large amount of food. While the stomach acid is busy with the big meal, the level of acid in the stomach drops, making it easier for bacteria like *Salmonella* to survive.

The major factor that determines whether or not you will become ill is how many bacteria you ingested. Hypothetically speaking, let us say that the skin of a chicken has 100,000 *Salmonella* bacteria on it. After you eat your chicken dinner and it enters the acidic environment of your stomach, 99% of the bacteria you have injested are killed. The stomach acid does an efficient job of killing the *Salmonella*, but in this case, there was a large initial number of bacteria that were ingested. If the initial numbers are lower, all of the *Salmonella* may be killed. However, in our hypothetical example, approximately 1,000 bacteria will still be left over. As you learned in Chapter 2, it only takes about 300 bacteria to make you sick.

SALMONELLA IN THE INTESTINES
Once swallowed, a mouthful of *Salmonella* enters the small intestine

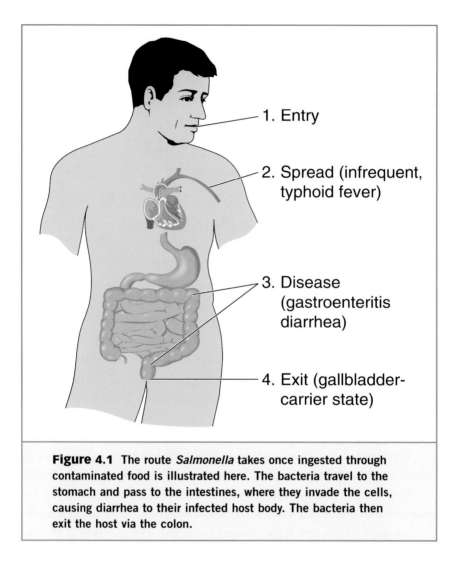

1. Entry

2. Spread (infrequent, typhoid fever)

3. Disease (gastroenteritis diarrhea)

4. Exit (gallbladder-carrier state)

Figure 4.1 The route *Salmonella* takes once ingested through contaminated food is illustrated here. The bacteria travel to the stomach and pass to the intestines, where they invade the cells, causing diarrhea to their infected host body. The bacteria then exit the host via the colon.

(Figure 4.1), where **microvilli**—finger-like projections designed to absorb water and nutrients—help protect the *Salmonella* that are not killed by the stomach acid (Figure 4.2). On the surface of the microvilli are cells, and it is these cells that the *Salmonella* invade. After they invade these cells, the bacteria start to multiply. Once *Salmonella* has entered a cell, the cell dies in about two hours. As the cell dies, it bursts open,

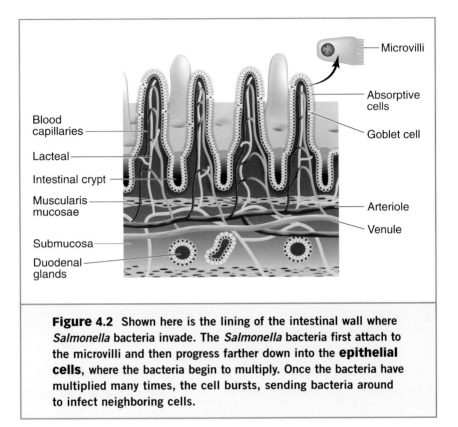

Figure 4.2 Shown here is the lining of the intestinal wall where *Salmonella* bacteria invade. The *Salmonella* bacteria first attach to the microvilli and then progress farther down into the **epithelial cells**, where the bacteria begin to multiply. Once the bacteria have multiplied many times, the cell bursts, sending bacteria around to infect neighboring cells.

spreading all of the *Salmonella* that just multiplied to surrounding cells, and the process starts over again. *Salmonella* enters the rest of the intestinal tract and is then excreted in the stool. As this cycle of invasion and cell destruction repeats, millions of bacteria are produced in the intestine, and their numbers continue to grow exponentially.

This cycle of invasion and destruction does not work entirely in the bacteria's favor, however. When a cell dies, it releases chemical signals that indicate that the cell is in distress. These chemical signals tell the body to start an immune reaction to the invading bacteria. Cells called **macrophages**—the immune system's primary response—seek out and engulf the bacteria to destroy them. The best way to picture how a macrophage works is to relate it to the video game Pac-Man®, where Pac-Man® goes around gobbling up all the foreign matter he encounters.

Like all other organisms, bacteria's main goal is to survive. To avoid being destroyed, *Salmonella* bacteria release a chemical that counteracts and disables the macrophages. Once this chemical is released, the invaded cell's chemical signal and the destroyed macrophages become part of the fluid that flows into the intestinal tract (rather than being absorbed). This results in diarrhea.

The intestines are lined with microvilli that can harbor *Salmonella* and help it enter epithelial cells of the intestines. An epithelial cell is a type of cell that covers most of the internal organs and many of the internal and external surfaces of the body. To enter the epithelial cells of the intestines, *Salmonella* bacteria use a spear- or needle-like projection to inject proteins directly into the epithelial cell. This needle-like structure is called a type III secretion apparatus. The proteins that are injected cause the epithelial cell to ruffle, like when you fluff sheets or blankets and they feather out, and ingest the *Salmonella*. The process of *Salmonella* entering the epithelial cell is often referred to as the "splash effect," because when the cell membrane does this ruffling, it looks like water rippling after a

SECRETION SYSTEMS

Bacteria have four secretion systems: type I, type II, type III, and type IV. Type I secretes the protein from the cytoplasm to directly outside the bacteria cell wall and then into the area of the host cell membrane where it enters. Type II secretes proteins into the periplasm and then transfers the proteins to the host cell membrane. Type III, which is found in *Salmonella*, transfers proteins from the bacteria across the cell membrane. Type IV codes for **pili** production and sends effector molecules from the bacteria to the cell surface.

stone is thrown into it. Once the bacteria are in the cell, they form **vacuoles** (small pockets of space). The vacuoles formed by *Salmonella* are specially designed to protect the bacteria from **lysosomes**, which are sack-like structures found inside most cells that contain chemicals designed to kill bacteria and dissolve materials that enter the cell. Once inside the vacuole, *Salmonella* bacteria are free to multiply (Figure 4.3).

THE BODY'S RESPONSE TO A *SALMONELLA* INVASION

Once *Salmonella* bacteria start to kill the cells of the infected person or animal (called the host), the dying cells send out distress signals in an effort to start an immune response. To counter this, *Salmonella* releases its own chemical, which neutralizes the macrophages sent by the body to attack the invading bacteria. In the battle between *Salmonella* and macrophages, bacteria, dead cells, chemical signals, and extra fluid build up eventually reaches the intestines of the infected person. It is only when these materials reach the intestines that the infected person realizes he or she is sick.

To flush the infection from the system, the body produces diarrhea, which may be bloody because of the lesions (sores) that are being made by the larger amount of fluids leaving the intestinal tract, and the body trying to defend itself against the bacteria that are invading the surrounding tissue. Cells in the body also release **cytokines**, a type of protein that activates and regulates the immune system. One of the body's main ways to fight an infection is fever, which raises the body temperature to try to kill the bacteria. A certain type of cytokine (IL-1) starts the **pyrogenic**, or fever-producing, response. Most invading bacteria are shed with the continuing diarrhea. The body's immune response—which includes macrophages, fever, and **antibodies** (proteins produced by the body to attack and destroy foreign materials)—kills the remaining bacteria.

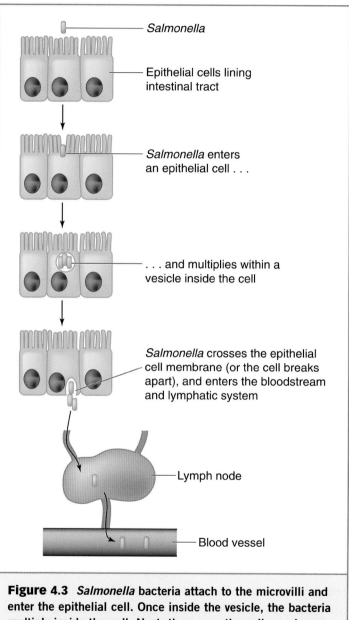

Salmonella

Epithelial cells lining
intestinal tract

Salmonella enters
an epithelial cell . . .

. . . and multiplies within a
vesicle inside the cell

Salmonella crosses the epithelial
cell membrane (or the cell breaks
apart), and enters the bloodstream
and lymphatic system

Lymph node

Blood vessel

Figure 4.3 *Salmonella* bacteria attach to the microvilli and
enter the epithelial cell. Once inside the vesicle, the bacteria
multiply inside the cell. Next, they cross the cell membrane
and enter the bloodstream and the lymphatic system before
ending up in a blood vessel.

Since the disease caused by *Salmonella* often runs its course naturally without forcing the infected person to seek medical assistance, it is often called **self-limiting**. Most cases of salmonellosis go away on their own in about 5 to 7 days. Only in severe cases—where the immune system cannot bring the bacteria down to a low enough level to be shed and destroyed—is antibiotic therapy needed. In such cases, doctors need to evaluate the illness and the patient's general state of health to determine what kind of treatment is the best. Various treatment options are discussed in Chapter 5.

5

Treating Salmonellosis

Most cases of salmonellosis are self-limiting. Severe cases, however, may require antibiotic treatment and rehydration therapy—especially if the patient has a weakened immune system. Rehydration therapy is used to replace fluids that are lost from diarrhea. The therapy involves ingesting fluids containing glucose and electrolytes (chemicals such as sodium and potassium). Sports drinks such as Gatorade® and the children's version of Pedialyte® are two such fluids that can be used to rehydrate patients. If this treatment is not sought soon enough and the patient goes to the doctor or emergency room, they will likely receive rehydration therapy intravenously (administered directly into a vein). The antibiotics that are most often prescribed for *Salmonella* infections are ampicillin, gentamicin, trimethoprim/sulfamethoxazole, or ciprofloxacin. There are many different choices of antibiotics because not all people are able to take the same kind of antibiotic and because several types of *Salmonella* have become resistant to antibiotics.

Antibiotics were first used in the 1940s to fight bacterial infections and they were a major medical breakthrough. Although antibiotics were not used widely until the 1940s, they were actually discovered much earlier by a French medical student named Ernest Duchesne, in 1896. He was the first person to learn about the antibiotic properties of the *Penicillium* mold, which is used for the antibiotic penicillin. However, the young doctor was unaware of what he had found and failed to notice that when this fungus was present, bacteria did not grow. His work was rediscovered when, in 1928, British bacteriologist Sir Alexander Fleming (Figure 5.1) made the same discovery that would forever change the medical world. Today, there are many antibiotics available to treat bacterial infections.

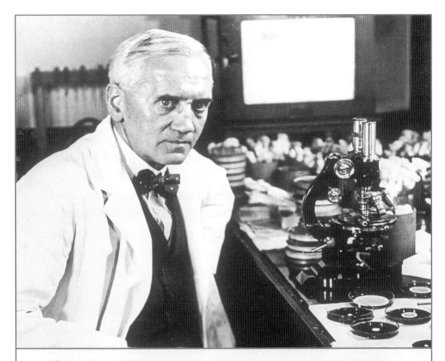

Figure 5.1 British bacteriologist Sir Alexander Fleming (shown here) is considered the father of antibiotic treatment. Fleming's 1928 discovery of penicillin came quite by accident during his research on influenza (the virus that causes the flu). He was growing bacterial plates in the lab when he noticed mold contamination on some of the plates. He thought all was lost due to the contamination, but then he noticed that no bacteria grew within a range around the mold. The mold he identified on the plate was *Penicillium* and the substance purified from it is known today as the antibiotic penicillin.

It is important to understand that there are two main groups of antibiotics: bactericidal and bacteriostatic. *Bactericidal* means "to destroy bacteria." There are three different categories of bactericidal agents: penicillins, cephalosporins, and aminoglycosides. Penicillins work by interfering with cell wall synthesis (the protective layer around the bacteria). Cephalosporins are broad-spectrum antibiotics that are effective against many different kinds of bacteria. This category can be differentiated into three groups: 1st, 2nd, and 3rd generation cephalosporins. Examples of 1st generation cephalosporins are cephazolin and cephalexin; 2nd generation members include cefuroxime and cefaclor, and 3rd generation cephalosporins include cefotaxime and ceftizoxime. The third category of bactericidal antibiotics is called aminoglycosides. These kill the bacteria by attaching to the **ribosome** and preventing the cells from misreading **RNA**. Some examples of aminoglycosides are gentamicin, streptomycin, and neomycin.

The second group of antibiotics, the bacteriostatic, work by inhibiting the growth and multiplication of the bacteria, which gives the host time to start an immune response to the bacteria. Some examples of bacteriostatic agents include sulphonamides, tetracyclines, chloramphenicol, erythromycin, and trimethoprim.

The antibiotics that are effective against salmonellosis are gentamycin, trimethoprim/sulfamethoxazole, ciprofloxacin, ampicillin, and tetracycline. As you can see, there is a wide range of antibiotics available to treat bacterial diseases such as salmonellosis. The most commonly used to combat *Salmonella* come from the penicillins, cephalosporins, and aminoglycosides— the bactericidal group, as well as some from the bacteriostatic group. However, antibiotics are only administered in severe cases of salmonellosis. Many of these antibiotics may soon be ineffective against salmonellosis because there are many strains of *Salmonella* appearing nationwide that are resistant to more than one antibiotic.

THE PROBLEM OF ANTIBIOTIC RESISTANCE

The use of antibiotics is sometimes necessary to kill bacteria that cause severe infections. However, the use of antibiotics— and especially the *overuse* of antibiotics—also causes a longer-term problem called **antibiotic resistance**, which occurs when a pathogen develops the ability to destroy or remain unaffected by a drug used against it.

The main goal of bacteria is to survive. When confronted with something that threatens their survival, bacteria—like any other living organism—do whatever they need to do to avoid or defeat the threat. When that threat is a chemical, an antibiotic for example, the bacteria must change themselves so that they are no longer affected by the chemical. We will discuss how antibiotic resistance occurs shortly. When bacteria mutate, the result is a "new and improved" version of the bacteria. No longer threatened by the antibiotic used to fight them, the bacteria are able to multiply and cause future infections.

Sometimes, bacteria become resistant to antibiotics simply because they already carry a gene for resistance. A **gene** is a structure in the cells of all living things that holds information about the organism's physical characteristics and functions;

KEEP TRACK OF YOUR HEALTH

It is a good idea for you to keep a record of your own health at home. The types of things you should enter in your health journal include any condition you have had and been treated for—for example, if you had strep throat and were treated by a doctor who gave you antibiotics. Write down the name of the antibiotic, how long you took it, and how your body reacted—for example, if you had any side effects like nausea, headache, appetite loss, or diarrhea. Diarrhea from an antibiotic is a normal side effect, since the medication is eliminating all of your normal bacterial flora as well as the disease-causing bacteria you are trying to kill. Keeping track of your ailments may help your doctor in the future decide which is the best antibiotic for you. It is also a good way to remember any antibiotics or drugs to which you are allergic. You are the best source of knowledge about what is going on with your body. Keeping a health journal will save you time and will help you live a safer, healthier life.

it is the basic unit of heredity. In general, there are three ways for bacteria to acquire genes for resistance to an antibiotic (Figure 5.2). The first is a **spontaneous mutation**, which is a sudden, natural change in the genetic makeup of an organism. In a spontaneous mutation, the **deoxyribonucleic acid (DNA)**— the chemical inside living cells that carries the organism's genetic information—suddenly changes. The change is often random and accidental, and is usually the result of a small error that the body makes while processing and producing its DNA.

A second way that bacteria can obtain genes for resistance is called **transformation**, commonly referred to as bacterial sex. In transformation, DNA from one bacterium is taken up by another bacterium. The process occurs when a bacterium picks up loose DNA that is coming out of another bacterial cell that has ruptured (split open).

The third way that bacteria obtain genes for resistance is probably the most efficient method for the bacteria, but the most difficult for researchers to study and fight. In this process, antibiotic resistance is obtained from a **plasmid**, or small circle of DNA. The difference between DNA and a plasmid is that DNA contains all of an organism's genetic information, whereas a plasmid is a small independent DNA molecule that only encodes the information for a few specific genes. Bacteria can transfer plasmids among themselves just by being close to one another. A bacterium that has plasmids carrying resistance genes can transfer its plasmids—and, therefore, its resistance— to another bacterium, even if the two bacteria are of completely different types. In Guatemala in 1968, 12,500 people died from a bacterium called *Shigella* because it harbored several plasmids that made it resistant to four antibiotics that were normally used for treatment.

Currently, many bacteria that cause infections are becoming resistant to antibiotics. This growing resistance is a major concern to the Centers for Disease Control and Prevention (CDC), microbiologists, and physicians. If this trend continues,

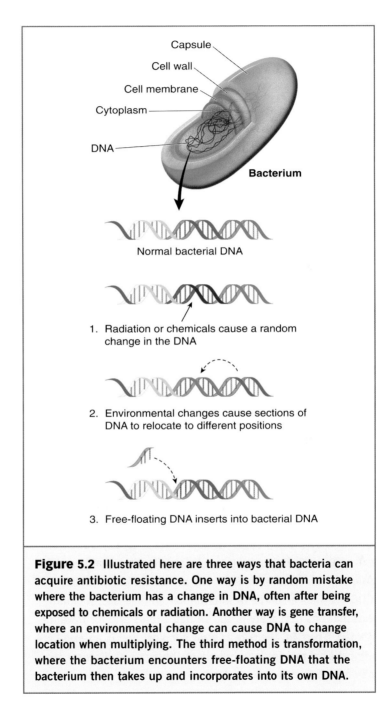

Figure 5.2 Illustrated here are three ways that bacteria can acquire antibiotic resistance. One way is by random mistake where the bacterium has a change in DNA, often after being exposed to chemicals or radiation. Another way is gene transfer, where an environmental change can cause DNA to change location when multiplying. The third method is transformation, where the bacterium encounters free-floating DNA that the bacterium then takes up and incorporates into its own DNA.

we will eventually reach a point at which we do not have any antibiotics that can effectively fight infections. This will be particularly dangerous for children, elderly people, and people who are prone to infections. It is not easy to develop an antibiotic that will be effective, and even antibiotics that show promise have to go through rigorous testing by the FDA before they can be given to patients. This process can take up to 10 years!

PREVENTING ANTIBIOTIC RESISTANCE

It is not possible to stop antibiotic resistance entirely. One of the biggest factors contributing to the growth of antibiotic resistance is the overuse of antibiotics by physicians. When a doctor prescribes an antibiotic for a patient who has an

WHAT IS THE CDC?

The CDC (Centers for Disease Control and Prevention) is a federal agency headquartered in Atlanta, Georgia. The CDC is responsible for the health and safety concerns of all citizens in the United States as well as American citizens traveling abroad. The agency monitors safety issues regarding health, such as reporting outbreaks of diseases, and environmental health issues as well, such as pollution as it relates to asthma. The CDC keeps strict records detailing all health outbreaks within the United States as well as those in other countries that may potentially affect the United States, for example the avian (bird) flu that started in Asia was a concern here in the United States when cases started to occur locally. Another example is the mosquito-borne West Nile virus that began in Asia and has steadily made its way across the United States. The CDC provides a source of information on diseases, including vaccinations necessary in the United States and for traveling abroad. The CDC Website is www.cdc.gov, and is an excellent educational tool for learning about the types of diseases that can affect your health.

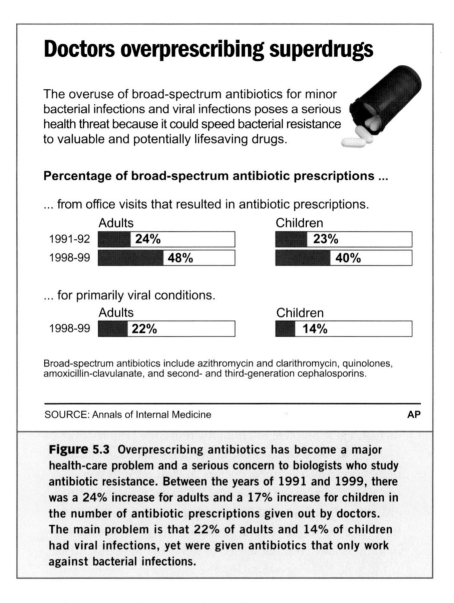

Doctors overprescribing superdrugs

The overuse of broad-spectrum antibiotics for minor bacterial infections and viral infections poses a serious health threat because it could speed bacterial resistance to valuable and potentially lifesaving drugs.

Percentage of broad-spectrum antibiotic prescriptions ...

... from office visits that resulted in antibiotic prescriptions.

	Adults	Children
1991-92	24%	23%
1998-99	48%	40%

... for primarily viral conditions.

	Adults	Children
1998-99	22%	14%

Broad-spectrum antibiotics include azithromycin and clarithromycin, quinolones, amoxicillin-clavulanate, and second- and third-generation cephalosporins.

SOURCE: Annals of Internal Medicine   AP

Figure 5.3 Overprescribing antibiotics has become a major health-care problem and a serious concern to biologists who study antibiotic resistance. Between the years of 1991 and 1999, there was a 24% increase for adults and a 17% increase for children in the number of antibiotic prescriptions given out by doctors. The main problem is that 22% of adults and 14% of children had viral infections, yet were given antibiotics that only work against bacterial infections.

infection caused by something other than a bacterium—say, for example, a virus—the resistance problem is worsened. Viruses are not killed by antibiotics, but any bacteria in the body, including beneficial bacteria, can be triggered to build up resistance to the antibiotic given (Figure 5.3).

The restrictions insurance companies put on doctors in terms of what tests they can run and what drugs they can prescribe further limits doctors' ability to help their patients. Some health insurance will only cover generic drugs instead of brand-name drugs, or will only give a price break for certain drugs. The result is that some doctors prescribe an antibiotic that is not the best one to fight the infection, but rather the only one that will meet the requirements of the patient's insurance company. The antibiotic may not be the best one available to kill a particular bacterium.

Allergies to antibiotics are another reason why some bacteria are developing resistance. When a patient is allergic to the best antibiotic available to fight his or her infection, a doctor may have to prescribe an antibiotic that is less effective.

Bacteria are also becoming resistant to antibiotics because many animals used for food, such as cattle and chicken, are given feed that contains antibiotics while they are being raised on the farm. The farmers want to keep their animals as healthy as possible so they fatten up and bring more money when they go to slaughter. As you saw in Chapter 3, animals play a major role as a source of *Salmonella* infection in people, a role that is increasing the problem of antibiotic resistance (Figure 5.4).

Finally, when patients fail to finish the full course of antibiotics prescribed by their doctors to treat an infection, they are contributing to the problem of antibiotic resistance. This is an extremely serious problem. In Chapter 1, Michelle's doctor instructed her to take ciprofloxacin for 7 days to cure her case of salmonellosis, but she started to feel better after just 3 days. If Michelle had stopped taking the antibiotics after the third day, the number of *Salmonella* bacteria in her body may have dropped low enough that she no longer showed symptoms of her infection, but some bacteria might still have been present. When this happens, the bacteria have time to multiply and cause another infection. The bacteria may also be able to mutate and become resistant to the prescribed antibiotic,

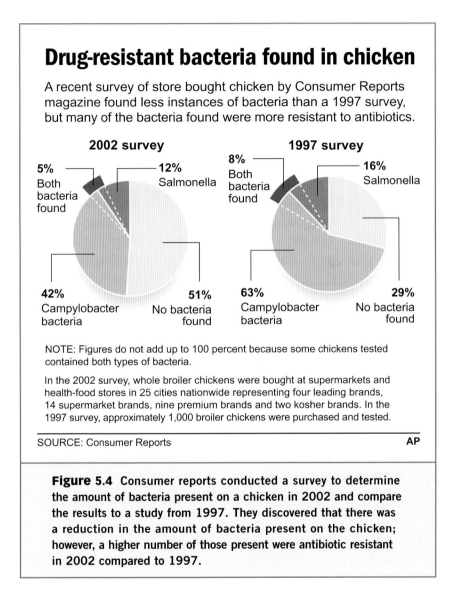

Drug-resistant bacteria found in chicken

A recent survey of store bought chicken by Consumer Reports magazine found less instances of bacteria than a 1997 survey, but many of the bacteria found were more resistant to antibiotics.

2002 survey

5% Both bacteria found

12% Salmonella

42% Campylobacter bacteria

51% No bacteria found

1997 survey

8% Both bacteria found

16% Salmonella

63% Campylobacter bacteria

29% No bacteria found

NOTE: Figures do not add up to 100 percent because some chickens tested contained both types of bacteria.

In the 2002 survey, whole broiler chickens were bought at supermarkets and health-food stores in 25 cities nationwide representing four leading brands, 14 supermarket brands, nine premium brands and two kosher brands. In the 1997 survey, approximately 1,000 broiler chickens were purchased and tested.

SOURCE: Consumer Reports   AP

Figure 5.4 Consumer reports conducted a survey to determine the amount of bacteria present on a chicken in 2002 and compare the results to a study from 1997. They discovered that there was a reduction in the amount of bacteria present on the chicken; however, a higher number of those present were antibiotic resistant in 2002 compared to 1997.

which would mean that Michelle could not take ciprofloxacin again to fight the infection. Whenever your doctor prescribes antibiotics, always be sure to complete the entire regimen and never skip doses. Otherwise, you, too, will be contributing to the dangerous problem of antibiotic resistance.

6

Salmonella Outbreaks and Current Research

In recent years, an increasing number of salmonellosis outbreaks have occurred around the world. Taking a closer look at a few of these outbreaks can help us better understand how common and how real a problem *Salmonella* is.

1. May 2002, Germany: Two hundred people became ill with salmonellosis after eating black forest cakes, pastries, and cannoli that had come in contact with raw egg products because a baker failed to wash his hands properly.

2. September 2002, England: One hundred fifty people became ill and two people died after eating eggs that were contaminated with *Salmonella*. The eggs had been purchased at different stores, but came from the same farm. The farm was issued citations on several health violations.

3. March 2003, Washington and Oregon: Several workers at an alfalfa sprout farm in Washington State became ill. The seeds that the workers had been handling were contaminated with *Salmonella*, which caused people working with them to become ill. In this case, the outbreak was localized among the plant workers who had been handling the contaminated seeds.

4. June 2003, Gates, New York: One hundred people fell ill after eating from the buffet at a wedding reception held at a golf club. The

particular food that caused the outbreak was not identified, but several of the items in the buffet were foods that
are likely sources of *Salmonella*: chicken breasts, egg
salad, dinner salad, and pastries. *Salmonella* was isolated
from several of the guests.

5. October 2003: A beef-processing plant in New Mexico
voluntarily recalled 22,000 pounds of beef jerky. An
inspection by the United States Department of Agriculture
(USDA) revealed that the contamination of the meat may
have been linked to an outbreak of salmonellosis in more
than 20 people who consumed the beef jerky. All beef
jerky that was produced between May and September 2003
was recalled.

These are only a few of the outbreaks that have been
recorded in the last few years. However, during the 1990s, there
were numerous outbreaks yearly around the world, and probably more cases that were not detected or reported. It is not
always easy to track infections with salmonellosis or other
infectious diseases in developing countries, nor do we know
the extent of food poisoning cases in the United States because
there are so many unreported or undocumented cases.

In 1996, the CDC developed SODA (*Salmonella* Outbreak
Detection Algorithm), a computer program designed to help
scientists detect clusters of *Salmonella* outbreaks that might
otherwise go unnoticed. SODA enables scientists to identify
infection sources more quickly and, hopefully, to prevent or
limit cases of the disease. PHLIS (the Public Health Laboratory
Information System), another computer program used by the
CDC, also tracks all outbreaks.

SALMONELLA RESEARCH

The CDC, NIH (National Institutes of Health), USDA, and
Food and Drug Administration (FDA) fund many projects
every year to help research groups that are studying *Salmonella*.

Current research projects include **sequencing**—determining the arrangement of the DNA that makes up the genes—of the different forms of *Salmonella*. Several forms of the bacterium, including one called *Salmonella typhimurium*, have already been sequenced, but most forms have not.

Every gene that is identified in the DNA sequence provides scientists with a better understanding of how *Salmonella* functions. Different DNA sequences **encode**, or provide the genetic instructions for, different features of the bacterium. Researchers have found sequences in other types of bacteria that encode for such features as **virulence**, **attachment**, antibiotic resistance, and toxin production. Some of these sequences closely match the sequences found in *Salmonella*. Sometimes, researchers identify genes but are not sure what they encode for. When this happens, the researchers alter the gene and then look to see if the change affects the ability of the bacteria to survive and cause infection. This is often how scientists find out what newly identified genes actually do.

Another growing area of *Salmonella* research is the struggle to fully understand the process by which the bacterium causes disease—this is referred to as the **pathogenesis** of the bacterium. Scientists do not yet know all the genes that are responsible for allowing bacteria to survive inside the intestines of hosts. It is important for researchers to identify the genes responsible for pathogenesis, since determining how *Salmonella* grows and spreads may provide insight into new ways to help the body's immune system respond to infections faster. Perhaps it will someday even show us a way to make the bacteria harmless.

A technique that is widely used in *Salmonella* research is called pulsed-field gel electrophoresis (PFGE). This technique shows the DNA profile of the different types of *Salmonella*. The profile shows up as a series of bands; each strain of *Salmonella* has a unique pattern. This tool is particularly useful because it can be used to test DNA extracted from fecal samples

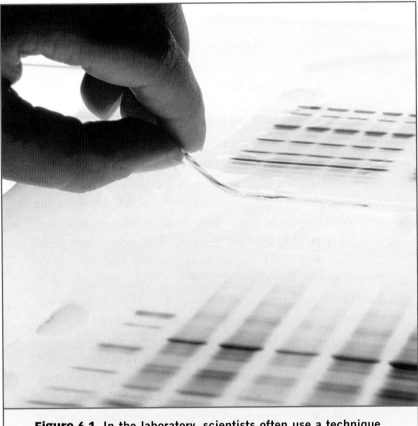

Figure 6.1 In the laboratory, scientists often use a technique called pulsed-field gel electrophoresis, which displays the DNA banding pattern of bacteria. This technique may be used to determine if several people who are sick with *Salmonella* are infected with the same strain. If the DNA bands are all identical, then all the patients are infected with the same strain and there is an outbreak that health officials need to investigate.

from people who get sick during a salmonellosis outbreak. PFGE can help determine the specific type of *Salmonella* that caused the outbreak. The CDC uses this method to track all outbreaks of salmonellosis (Figure 6.1).

Another new technique being used in *Salmonella* research is called real-time polymerase chain reaction (RT-PCR). In

RT-PCR, a fecal sample suspected of containing *Salmonella* is examined to see if it contains a certain sequence of DNA. If that DNA sequence is found, the sample is considered positive for *Salmonella*. This process reveals not only whether the sample is contaminated with *Salmonella*, but also how many *Salmonella* bacteria are present in the sample. RT-PCR is a handy test for finding out whether a food product has enough *Salmonella* present to make the people who eat it sick.

Many companies are also trying to create rapid detection kits that would test food products instantly for the presence of *Salmonella*. These products would work like litmus paper—the pH test strips we use to check the level of chlorine in a pool. These kits would be useful in restaurants, where they could help chefs and cooks prepare food properly and thus reduce the risk of food-borne illness.

Finally, another area of research is vaccine production. A **vaccine** is a drug made from a weakened or killed pathogen that stimulates the immune system to protect the body against the pathogen. A main area of focus is the development of a vaccine for use on farms that raise food animals, especially chickens. An effective vaccine against salmonellosis in chickens and cattle would provide significant economic benefits to farmers. A potential vaccine against salmonellosis in chickens has been developed but is still being studied.

A *SALMONELLA* VACCINE FOR HUMANS?

Currently, there is one vaccine that has been approved for use in chickens against a form of *Salmonella* called *Salmonella enteritidis*. This vaccine has not been approved for humans, however, and likely will not be in the near future due to the extensive testing that needs to be done by the FDA before any new vaccine is approved. Another vaccine against a form of *Salmonella* called *Salmonella typhi* has also been developed, but is only 60% effective. A person given this vaccine would still have a strong chance of developing salmonellosis.

SALMONELLA AS A BIOLOGICAL WEAPON

To assess the threat of bioterrorism, the CDC has established three different categories of seriousness. The first, category A, includes organisms that are easily spread from person to person, which will result in a high **mortality rate** and may cause panic among the population and require public health agencies and facilities to prepare for disease outbreaks. The pathogens in this category include those that cause plague, anthrax, botulism, smallpox, tularemia, and viral hemorrhagic fevers. The pathogens in category B are described as relatively easy to transfer from person to person, and will have a moderate level of mortality. They require the CDC to be prepared to quickly identify the pathogens involved and publish relevant information for the public and health-care officials. This is the largest group, with 15 pathogens. Some of the pathogens on this list are *Brucella*, *Clostridium perfringens*, *Shigella*, *Escherichia coli* O157:H7, and *Salmonella*. The third and final group is category C. This group includes emerging pathogens that are easy to obtain and transmit and can also cause high mortality. This group is the smallest, since most of the diseases are emerging; the only two listed are Nipah virus and hantavirus.

It is not likely that there will be a single vaccine that is effective against all the different forms of *Salmonella* anytime soon. As we learned in Chapter 1, there are more than 2,500 different types of *Salmonella* that can infect people. There is enough genetic variation between these types that it is not possible for a single a vaccine to work against all of them. Ongoing research is investigating what can be done to produce a useful human vaccine for *Salmonella*. Instead of waiting for a vaccine, however, there are steps you can take to help prevent salmonellosis yourself, which will be discussed in Chapter 8.

7

Other Bacteria That Cause Food Poisoning

The main focus of this book is *Salmonella*, but there are several other types of bacteria that cause food poisoning, including *Escherichia coli*, *Vibrio cholerae*, *Campylobacter jejuni*, *Listeria monocytogenes*, *Shigella*, *Staphylococcus aureus*, and *Yersinia enterocolitica*. These are only some of the more common causes of bacterial food poisoning; there are several hundred other types of bacteria that can contaminate food and cause illness in people. It is important that you are aware of some of the other common food-borne pathogens. Since reporting of these pathogens, including *Salmonella*, is not as accurate as it could be, being aware of just some of the many different food-borne illnesses that could infect you and how you could become infected (i.e., the different sources) with them will help your doctor with diagnosis and better surveillance. As you read this section, think about what you have learned about *Salmonella* and salmonellosis, and compare the similarities of the pathogens and diseases described here. You will notice that there is some overlap in the kinds of foods that can cause different food-borne diseases. Also, there are only slight variations in the symptoms of the different diseases. This is just to broaden your knowledge on some of the major pathogens that can be present in your food supply. When most people hear about a disease outbreak from food, they automatically assume it is either *Salmonella* or *E. coli* 0157:H7, but after reading the following you will understand how untrue that assumption can be.

ESCHERICHIA COLI O157:H7

When you hear about cases of food poisoning on the news, more often than not *Escherichia coli* O157:H7 is the cause. Every year, there are an estimated 73,000 cases of infection with this bacterium, causing about 61 deaths. This bacterium is not the only form of *Escherichia coli*—there are literally hundreds of others. Outbreaks of *Escherichia coli* O157:H7 infection were first recorded in 1982 when around 47 people became ill in Oregon and Michigan after eating tainted hamburgers at McDonald's® fast-food restaurants. The most notorious outbreak was in 1993 when 600 people became ill, and 4 children died from eating undercooked hamburgers from a Jack In The Box® restaurant in Washington State.

Infections with this organism most often result from eating undercooked or raw meat products, especially ground beef. Meat becomes contaminated with *Escherichia coli* O157:H7 during slaughter when the entrails are removed from the cattle, because the bacteria usually reside in the intestines. The bacterium may also be present on cow udders. Other sources of infection include sprouts, lettuce, salami, unpasteurized milk or juice, or bodies of water such as wading or swimming pools. The symptoms of *Escherichia coli* O157:H7 infection include abdominal cramps, severe bloody diarrhea, and possibly a fever. The symptoms last for 5 to 10 days and are usually self-limiting. If the symptoms persist, antibiotics may be prescribed. In severe cases, a condition called hemolytic uremic syndrome (HUS)—which is caused by a **toxin** produced by the bacteria—may develop. HUS can result in acute kidney failure. In such cases, patients need dialysis treatments for the rest of their lives. In extreme cases, kidney transplants may be needed. Infection with *Escherichia coli* O157:H7 can be prevented by cooking all meat thoroughly to a temperature of 140°F (60°C), and only drinking milk and juices that have been **pasteurized.**

VIBRIO CHOLERAE

Vibrio cholerae (Figure 7.1), the bacterium that causes a disease called cholera, affects only about 5 people each year in the United States, but it is widespread in many developing countries. Cholera is an acute diarrheal disease, contracted through drinking contaminated water. The risk of infection in the United States is low because almost all drinking water is treated and free of sewage. In developing countries, however, water is not as plentiful and is often not treated properly, especially after floods. In some countries, people use the same water for drinking, cooking, and bathing that animals drink and defecate in. This contaminates the water, passing infections from animals to people. Infections can also occur after eating shellfish that come from contaminated water.

The clinical signs of cholera are a profuse watery diarrhea, vomiting, and collapse of the circulatory system. The diarrhea is often referred to as rice water stool, since the stools are very watery and contain lots of mucus. There is a 25 to 50% **fatality rate** from cholera. The fatality rate is so high because the disease causes enormous fluid loss. It is very common for a person with cholera to lose 20 liters (21 quarts) of fluid in a single day. It is extremely difficult to rehydrate a person who has lost this much fluid. Even so, if fluid rehydration therapy is given quickly and consistently for the duration of the illness, fewer than 1% of patients die.

Americans who travel to developing countries are particularly susceptible to cholera. To prevent infection with *Vibrio cholerae*, a person traveling in a country where cholera is present should boil all water before drinking, bathing, or brushing his or her teeth. Ice should not be used unless it is made from water that has been boiled or treated. Only foods that have been thoroughly cooked should be eaten. All fruits should be peeled and all outside layers of the fruit should be discarded, since the skin of the fruit is the part most likely to have come into contact with contaminated water.

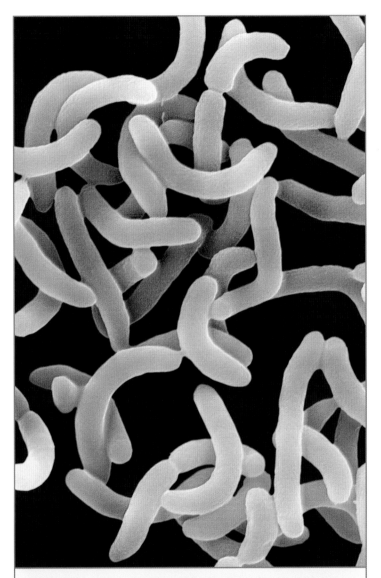

Figure 7.1 This scanning electron micrograph (magnified 2,500 times) depicts the long rod-shaped bacteria called *Vibrio cholerae* that is usually transmitted in contaminated water. When infected with these bacteria, you may lose up to 20 liters of water a day through diarrhea, making rehydration therapy very important.

CAMPYLOBACTER JEJUNI

Campylobacter jejuni (Figure 7.2) is the leading cause of bacterial food-borne illness in the United States. An estimated 2.4 million cases of *Campylobacter jejuni* infection, or campylobacteriosis, occur every year, with 124 of those cases being fatal.

Campylobacteriosis is characterized by abdominal cramps, severe bloody diarrhea, and fever that lasts for 2 to 5 days. Some cases also include nausea and vomiting. Occasionally, campylobacteriosis becomes systemic and life-threatening. In about 1 out of 1,000 cases, campylobacteriosis leads to a condition called Guillain-Barré syndrome, a paralysis that can last for weeks and often requires the patient to receive intensive care. It is estimated that 40% of all Guillain-Barré cases begin with a *Campylobacter jejuni* infection.

Campylobacteriosis occurs after a person eats under-cooked or raw poultry, meat, or pork, or milk products or juices that are unpasteurized. *Campylobacter jejuni* infections are usually self-limiting, but in severe cases, antibiotics may be needed. Over the past several years, *Campylobacter jejuni* has become resistant to many antibiotics. Rehydration therapy is the most common treatment for campylobacteriosis, with the use of **analgesics** for fever reduction. Campylobacteriosis can be prevented by washing and cooking all meats thoroughly and drinking only juices and milk products that have been pasteurized.

LISTERIA MONOCYTOGENES

The bacterium *Listeria monocytogenes* (Figure 7.3) is responsible for about 2,500 cases of food-borne illness per year, about 500 of which are fatal. Infection with *Listeria monocytogenes* (listeriosis) causes different problems for different groups of people. For instance, in people who are elderly or immuno-compromised, sepsis and meningitis (a swelling of the tissues surrounding the brain and spinal cord) are the main symptoms. Pregnant women normally experience symptoms such as aches,

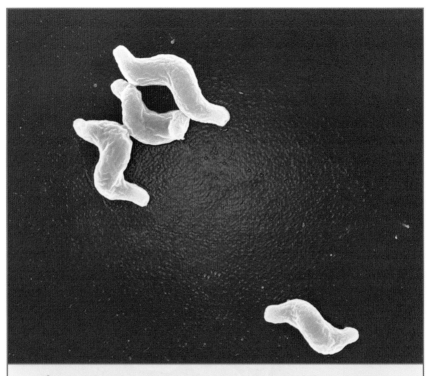

Figure 7.2 This scanning electron micrograph of *Campylobacter jejuni* (magnified 25,000 times) shows the curved rod shape of the bacterium. Campylobacteriosis is the leading cause of bacterial diarrheal disease in the world.

pains, stiff neck, confusion, and fever, followed by spontaneous abortion or meningitis in the fetus. In a healthy person, the disease causes acute gastroenteritis.

The main source of infection with *Listeria monocytogenes* is unpasteurized milk, although turkey and deli meats, especially packaged meats, can also cause infection. In several instances over the past few years, packaged meats have been recalled after being linked to outbreaks of listeriosis.

Infections have also been passed from person to person through **nosocomial transmission**, or hospital-acquired infection, although this is rare. People who are more susceptible to

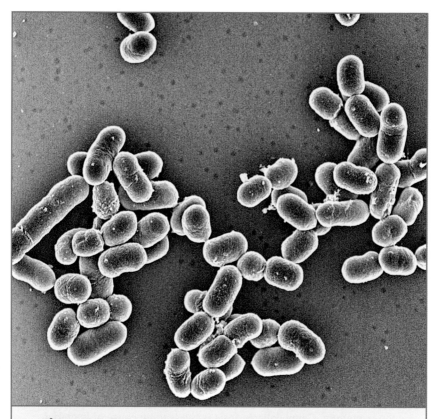

Figure 7.3 This scanning electron micrograph of *Listeria monocytogenes* shows the short, thick rod shape of the bacteria. This organism causes spontaneous abortion of the fetus in pregnant women and is often found in unpasteurized milk.

an infection with listeriosis are newborns, those with weakened immune systems, and persons with cancer, diabetes, or diseases of the kidney. A person with AIDS is 300 times more likely to contract listeriosis than is a person with a healthy immune system.

One of the unique characteristics of *Listeria* is that it can grow at refrigeration temperatures, whereas most bacteria need to be at room temperature or higher to reproduce. Listeriosis can be prevented by cooking all foods completely and drinking only pasteurized beverages. Pregnant women should avoid high-risk foods and handle all high-risk food products carefully. If the infection is detected immediately and prompt medical attention is sought, antibiotic therapy is available.

SHIGELLA

There are four different types of *Shigella* that cause food-borne illness: *Shigella boydii, Shigella dysenteriae, Shigella flexneri,* and *Shigella sonnei.* In the United States, there are about 450,000 annual cases of *Shigella* infection (shigellosis), 85% of which are caused by *Shigella sonnei.* In developing countries, *Shigella flexneri* is the type most commonly associated with infections in people.

Shigellosis is usually transmitted when material from the stool of a person with the disease ends up into contact with another person's mouth—often by way of water that has been improperly treated. This is referred to as the fecal-oral route, and is often a problem in areas where hygiene practices, sanitation, and sewage treatment are poor. Illness can easily occur if people who handle food products do not wash their hands properly after using the restroom. *Shigella* is also carried by flies, which often land on fecal matter (such as dog droppings) and then land on food. Groups that are at higher risk of infection include elderly people, travelers, and small children—especially children in group day-care settings, since children often lack proper hygiene habits.

Shigellosis is characterized by watery or bloody diarrhea, abdominal pain, fever, and **malaise**. One of the factors that makes this disease so easy to spread is the small number of bacteria needed to cause infection. As few as 10 bacteria can cause infection in a person, compared with *Salmonella,* which needs 300 organisms to be present to cause disease. A person with shigellosis usually recovers within a week or two, but in rare cases, it may take several months before the sufferer's bowel movements return to normal. About 3% of people with shigellosis develop a condition called Reiter's syndrome, which is characterized by joint pain, irritation of the eyes, and painful urination.

Shigellosis can be treated with antibiotics such as ampicillin or ciprofloxacin. Antidiarrheal agents such as Imodium or Pepto-Bismol are likely to increase the symptoms of the disease and should be avoided. Shigellosis does not have a cure and has to run its course and be eliminated from the body. By taking antidiarrheal agents, you are preventing your body from ridding itself of the bacteria and are keeping the bacteria inside you, where it will continue to make you sick over and over. Shigellosis can be prevented by proper handwashing when handling foods and cooking foods properly.

STAPHYLOCOCCUS AUREUS

Staphylococcus aureus (Figure 7.4) is responsible for approximately 100,000 cases of food poisoning every year. With

FOOD POISONING IN DEVELOPING COUNTRIES

Bacterial infections such as those discussed in this chapter are a common cause of food-borne disease. However, in developing countries, parasitic infections are much more prevalent than bacterial infections. This is important to you as a traveler, since many people who live in developing countries are carriers of parasites, simply because the parasites are so common. This stems from the lack of water sanitation and proper sewage systems. Some of the most common parasitic infections are filarial worms, tapeworm, *Leishmania*, *Giardia*, *Cryptosporidium*, *Schistosoma*, *Cyclospora*, flukes, and amoebas. These parasitic infections often cause the same symptoms as bacterial infections: diarrhea, fever, abdominal cramping, and dehydration. If you are traveling to a developing country, it is important to keep this in mind and take steps to protect yourself from infection.

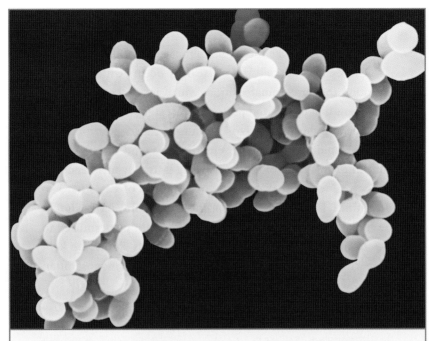

Figure 7.4 *Staphylococcus aureus* (shown here in an image taken with a scanning electron microscope and magnified 3,025 times) is often referred to as the "cluster of grapes" bacteria. This is due to the way the bacteria arrange themselves in clusters, as seen here.

Staphylococcus, the threat to health is more the result of toxins created by the bacterium than of the infection itself.

Infection with *Staphylococcus* is characterized by symptoms of severe diarrhea, vomiting, fever, aches, and abdominal cramping that may last up to three days. The effects of *Staphylococcus* infection are violent because the toxin produced by the bacteria once inside the body is powerful. The toxin attacks the **vagus nerve**, which controls the vomiting response. Several foods are possible sources of *Staphylococcus*, including meat, poultry, eggs, tuna or potato salad prepared with mayonaise, cream-filled pastries, cream pies, and dairy products. *Staphylococcus* is often referred to as the "picnic disease," since many common picnic foods—such as potato salad, coleslaw, and pies—are eaten after being left unrefrigerated, which gives the bacteria time to multiply and emit the toxin that causes sickness.

Disease from *Staphylococcus* usually occurs within 6 hours of eating the contaminated food, which is quicker than most pathogens that cause food poisoning. Most food-borne diseases can take anywhere from 6 to 72 hours to cause infections. The disease rapidly produces severe diarrhea and simultaneous vomiting. This form of food poisoning is usually misdiagnosed as the flu, which makes the actual number of cases hard to determine. To prevent *Staphylococcus* infections, foods should be cooked properly, creamy foods should not be permitted to sit out at room temperature, and cold foods should be kept properly refrigerated. *Staphylococcus* infection is most often treated with fluid replacement therapy.

YERSINIA ENTEROCOLITICA

About 500,000 cases of food poisoning each year are attributed to *Yersinia enterocolitica*. Infection with *Yersinia* (yersiniosis) is characterized by fever, abdominal pain, and bloody diarrhea that can last from 4 days to 3 weeks. This disease is most often seen in children and young adults. In young adults and adults, the disease causes severe pain on the side of the body and is often misdiagnosed as appendicitis. The most common source of yersiniosis is undercooked pork products, as well as unpasteurized milk. Most cases are self-limiting and do not lead to long-term problems. However, there are rare cases where pain in the knees, ankles, or wrists develops and lasts for 1 to 6 months. Antibiotics such as fluoroquinolones can be used for treatment but they are rarely given, since the disease usually goes away on its own.

Another source of infection is the fecal-oral route. This is particularly common in day-care centers, since young children do not always practice proper hygiene and can pass the infection to each other. To prevent infection with *Yersinia enterocolitica*, people should thoroughly cook all pork products and use proper hygiene when handling food products.

As you probably realize, this chapter deviated slightly from the main focus of this book, *Salmonella*. But think about everything you have just learned about *Salmonella* and compare it to the information about the organisms you just read about. Do you see a lot of common features among the different organisms? You should notice that most of the symptoms are the same for infections caused by the different organisms, and that the kinds of foods that can cause disease are often similar. By understanding both *Salmonella* and the other types of food-borne pathogens, you can take steps to avoid getting sick.

8

Preventing Salmonellosis

EDUCATING PEOPLE

One of the best ways to prevent food-borne illness is to educate the public. If people become aware of how their actions can contribute to the prevention or spread of food-borne diseases, there will likely be fewer cases. However, this is no easy task. To reach every person with this important information is an ambitious and difficult challenge. One thing you can do to stay informed about the threat of food-borne illness is to visit your local public health department's Website and read about current outbreaks and what health officials are doing to stop and prevent them.

Farmers, day laborers, and other people who are involved in agriculture should be educated about sanitation principles and how to properly handle food items to minimize the risk of contaminating the products. Education costs money, however, and it can be difficult to find funding to educate the general population. You can help get the message out yourself by sharing what you have learned about *Salmonella* and other bacteria that cause food-borne illnes with others.

MEASURES GROCERY STORES CAN TAKE TO PROTECT US

All grocery stores and supermarkets must follow FDA requirements regarding shipping, storage, and display temperature. Stores are also regulated by local health departments, which perform health inspections, issue licenses, and—when stores violate food safety rules—charge fines. For example, health inspectors make sure refrigerators are at the appropriate temperatures for the food they are storing. The health department determines if stores are clean enough, and also checks to make sure there are not too many insects, which can carry disease-causing bacteria. Some stores have taken the precaution of adding blowers over all doorways that blow down a constant stream of air that deters insects from entering the stores. Some stores wash all produce before placing it in bins. Meat departments are required to date all meat when it comes in, and provide a second date by which the meat needs to be sold.

If you are interested in the procedures your local store uses to protect you from food-borne illnesses, ask the store manager: This is public information. You can ask to see the store's inspection records, which will reveal whether the store has had any violations. You can also get this information from your city health department's Website.

HOW RESTAURANTS CAN PREVENT FOOD-BORNE ILLNESS

Restaurants are the most common places people acquire *Salmonella* and other food-borne pathogens. If the chefs and cooks in a restaurant fail to handle and prepare food correctly in the kitchen—for instance, if employees leave meats, chicken, or foods that spoil easily out at room temperature—the risk of salmonellosis is increased. State health departments inspect restaurants, and a surprising and disturbing number of them fail their inspections and are temporarily closed. Restaurants that fail health inspections are required to implement new health measures before they can reopen. Again, you can check this information on your local or state health department's Website before you eat at a restaurant. Some newspapers publish this information monthly to help educate the public.

Restaurant employees are required to take a class, pass a test, and get a food handler's permit before they start serving food, which must be renewed every several years (this varies by state). The food handler's permit tests are taken at the state restaurant licensing center. The test consists of reading a manual on the proper techniques for handling all food, the proper storage temperature of all foods and what temperature each food item must be cooked to. This manual also talks about personal hygiene practices that must be used by everyone who handles food. You can always ask to see a restaurant's last inspection record and operation permit. A good rule of thumb when you go out to eat is to look around. If the eating area, tables, chairs, and workers look dirty, then the kitchen is probably dirty, too. It is always better to leave a restaurant if you have doubts about how clean it is.

PROTECTING YOURSELF AT HOME

Perhaps the easiest way you can help fight food-borne illnesses such as *Salmonella* is to practice proper food-handling techniques in your own home (Figure 8.1). How can you do this? The simplest way is by washing your hands. This does not mean sticking your fingers under running water for a couple of seconds and then wiping them on whatever towel is handy. The proper way to wash your hands is to wet your hands with hot water, apply soap, and then say the alphabet to yourself while you scrub your hands with the soapy lather. Reciting the alphabet ensures that you spend enough time getting your hands clean. After you finish the alphabet, you should rinse your hands with hot water and dry them on a clean towel, or, if necessary, a hot-air dryer. This simple act is extremely effective. A surprising number of people wash their hands improperly or—worse—not at all. The next time you are in a public restroom, watch how many people leave without washing their hands and how many just rinse their hands with water for a short time. Keep in mind that once you start watching out for this, you may be disgusted! One other technique that you may want to employ in a public restroom is to use a paper towel to open the door as you exit the restroom. If the person before you didn't wash his or her hands and just used the handle to open the door, the handle now has germs on it, and these will get on your hands when

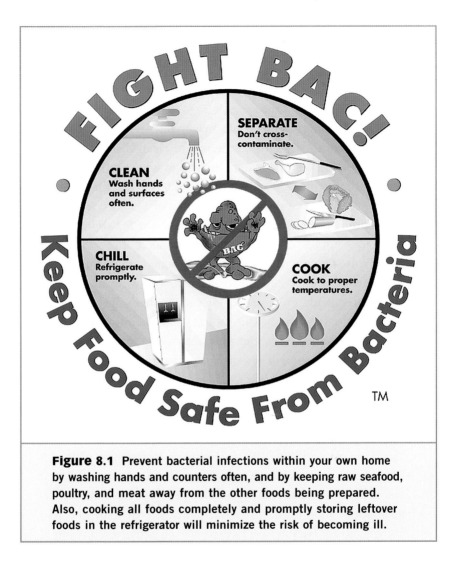

Figure 8.1 Prevent bacterial infections within your own home by washing hands and counters often, and by keeping raw seafood, poultry, and meat away from the other foods being prepared. Also, cooking all foods completely and promptly storing leftover foods in the refrigerator will minimize the risk of becoming ill.

you touch the door. This is another effective way you can help reduce your risk of illness.

A way to prevent food-borne illness in your kitchen is to avoid cross-contaminating food. For example, if you have just cut chicken on your cutting board, do not prepare the lettuce for a salad on the same cutting board. All cutting boards, knives, and bowls that come in contact with raw food should be washed with hot, soapy water. Make sure you wash all vegetables (except lettuce, just peel the outside layers off then rinse; recall Chapter 3) and fruits thoroughly.

Another item in many kitchens that has the potential to cause salmonellosis is the sponge. It may not occur to you that your dishwashing sponge could make you sick. Most people use a sponge to wipe off counters and clean dishes. If you cut up raw chicken and use the sponge to wipe up the juices, then wipe off the cutting board, should you use that same sponge to clean your dishes? No! If you have a kitchen sponge, make sure you only use it either for dishes or for wiping off counters—not both. Only use it on the counter after you have already used a paper towel with soapy water to wipe up any juices from poultry and meat. Make sure you replace your sponge frequently. You can prolong your sponge's life by filling it with water (i.e., wetting the sponge) and microwaving it on high for 2 minutes. Be careful when removing the sponge from the microwave, as it will be very hot.

Another common time for *Salmonella* to pose a threat is when you barbecue. For example, imagine you are at a picnic with your friend's family and you notice that the person who cooked the chicken brought the raw meat out on a platter and then later placed the cooked chicken back on the same platter. The cook just unwittingly cross-contaminated the chicken you are about to eat. This is your chance to share your knowledge about food-borne diseases. Remember that no one is going to speak for you; you have to take an active role in your own health.

When you are cooking, make sure you cook all foods completely. Chicken should not have any pink areas left in it. It is important to cook pork and beef thoroughly as well. Keep foods that need to be cold properly refrigerated. Any dairy products—for example, cheese, milk, and sour cream—should not be left out of the refrigerator for long. Do not leave the gallon of milk on the table throughout the meal; this just gives *Salmonella* and many other pathogens a chance to grow. If you are attending a picnic and will be outside in the heat, do not bring foods that will spoil easily, such as potato salad and coleslaw. These are traditional picnic foods, yet the fact is that many picnics have ended with guests running for the bathroom! These simple precautions can help make your special gathering both fun and safe.

Another way to prevent salmonellosis is to try to keep the doors to your house shut. If you have screen doors, make sure they do not have any holes in them. This will prevent insects, especially flies, from entering your house and contaminating your food. If you own pets, try to keep them away from cooking and eating areas. We all love our pets and consider them members of the family, but they can be the dirtiest members of the family and they can easily transmit salmonellosis to you. Children are very susceptible to infections with *Salmonella*, and pets can transfer the bacteria to children. Do not let your pet lick you, especially on your face. Make sure you wash your hands properly after playing with your pet and make sure your

SALMONELLOSIS FROM REPTILES

Los Angeles County in California has the most cases of salmonellosis yearly from reptiles. In the past ten years, there has been an increase in the number of green iguanas imported from Central America. In Los Angeles, these iguanas have become very popular pets and have a high rate of carrying *Salmonella* that then gets passed on to the pet owner and his or her family. Snakes have become more popular as pets in the last decade, as well. In order to decrease the number of cases of salmonellosis from reptiles, restrictions may need to be placed on the animals that are brought to the United States. So far, the only regulations are for turtles; other reptiles need to be monitored in similar ways.

pets are properly groomed. If you come across stray animals, try to handle them as little as possible, since you never know what kind of organisms they might be carrying.

The purpose of this book is not to scare you, but to educate you about the presence of *Salmonella* in your daily life. This text has provided you with information about what *Salmonella* is, where it can be found, how it infects you, how your body responds to the infection, and how you can help prevent salmonellosis. Hopefully, you will take what you have learned here and share it with others so that more people will understand the dangers of *Salmonella* and learn how infection can be avoided.

Centers for Disease Control and Prevention
Division of Bacterial and Mycotic Diseases
Disease Information: Salmonellosis

WHAT IS SALMONELLOSIS?

Salmonellosis is an infection with a bacteria called *Salmonella*. Most persons infected with *Salmonella* develop diarrhea, fever, and abdominal cramps 12 to 72 hours after infection. The illness usually lasts 4 to 7 days, and most persons recover without treatment. However, in some persons the diarrhea may be so severe that the patient needs to be hospitalized. In these patients, the *Salmonella* infection may spread from the intestines to the blood stream, and then to other body sites and can cause death unless the person is treated promptly with antibiotics. The elderly, infants, and those with impaired immune systems are more likely to have a severe illness.

WHAT SORT OF GERM IS *SALMONELLA*?

The *Salmonella* germ is actually a group of bacteria that can cause diarrheal illness in humans. They are microscopic living creatures that pass from the feces of people or animals, to other people or other animals. There are many different kinds of *Salmonella* bacteria. *Salmonella* serotype Typhimurium and *Salmonella* serotype Enteritidis are the most common in the United States. *Salmonella* has been known to cause illness for over 100 years. They were discovered by a American scientist named Salmon, for whom they are named.

HOW CAN *SALMONELLA* INFECTIONS BE DIAGNOSED?

Many different kinds of illnesses can cause diarrhea, fever, or abdominal cramps. Determining that *Salmonella* is the cause of the illness depends on laboratory tests that identify *Salmonella* in the stools of an infected person. These tests are sometimes not performed unless the laboratory is instructed specifically to look for the organism. Once *Salmonella* has been identified, further testing can determine its specific type, and which antibiotics could be used to treat it.

HOW CAN *SALMONELLA* INFECTIONS BE TREATED?

Salmonella infections usually resolve in 5–7 days and often do not require treatment unless the patient becomes severely dehydrated or the infection spreads from the intestines. Persons with severe diarrhea may require rehydration, often with intravenous fluids. Antibiotics are not usually necessary unless the infection spreads from the intestines, then it can be treated with ampicillin, gentamicin, trimethoprim/sulfamethoxazole, or ciprofloxacin. Unfortunately, some *Salmonella* bacteria have become resistant to antibiotics, largely as a result of the use of antibiotics to promote the growth of feed animals.

ARE THERE LONG-TERM CONSEQUENCES TO A *SALMONELLA* INFECTION?

Persons with diarrhea usually recover completely, although it may be several months before their bowel habits are entirely normal. A small number of persons who are infected with *Salmonella*, will go on to develop pains in their joints, irritation of the eyes, and painful urination. This is called Reiter's syndrome. It can last for months or years, and can lead to chronic arthritis which is difficult to treat. Antibiotic treatment does not make a difference in whether or not the person later develops arthritis.

HOW DO PEOPLE CATCH *SALMONELLA*?

Salmonella live in the intestinal tracts of humans and other animals, including birds. *Salmonella* are usually transmitted to humans by eating foods contaminated with animal feces. Contaminated foods usually look and smell normal. Contaminated foods are often of animal origin, such as beef, poultry, milk, or eggs, but all foods, including vegetables may become contaminated. Many raw foods of animal origin are frequently contaminated, but fortunately, thorough cooking kills *Salmonella*. Food may also become contaminated by the unwashed hands of an infected food handler, who forgot to wash his or her hands with soap after using the bathroom.

Salmonella may also be found in the feces of some pets, especially those with diarrhea, and people can become infected if they do not wash their hands after contact with these feces. Reptiles are particularly likely to harbor *Salmonella* and people should always wash their hands immediately after handling a reptile, even if the reptile is healthy. Adults should also be careful that children wash their hands after handling a reptile.

WHAT CAN A PERSON DO TO PREVENT THIS ILLNESS?

There is no vaccine to prevent salmonellosis. Since foods of animal origin may be contaminated with *Salmonella*, people should not eat raw or undercooked eggs, poultry, or meat. Raw eggs may be unrecognized in some foods such as homemade hollandaise sauce, caesar and other homemade salad dressings, tiramisu, homemade ice cream, homemade mayonnaise, cookie dough, and frostings. Poultry and meat, including hamburgers, should be well-cooked, not pink in the middle. Persons also should not consume raw or unpasteurized milk or other dairy products. Produce should be thoroughly washed before consuming.

Cross-contamination of foods should be avoided. Uncooked meats should be keep separate from produce, cooked foods, and ready-to-eat foods. Hands, cutting boards, counters, knives, and other utensils should be washed thoroughly after handling uncooked foods. Hand should be washed before handling any food, and between handling different food items.

People who have salmonellosis should not prepare food or pour water for others until they have been shown to no longer be carrying the *Salmonella* bacterium.

People should wash their hands after contact with animal feces. Since reptiles are particularly likely to have *Salmonella*, everyone should immediately wash their hands after handling reptiles. Reptiles (including turtles) are not appropriate pets for small children and should not be in the same house as an infant.

HOW COMMON IS SALMONELLOSIS?

Every year, approximately 40,000 cases of salmonellosis are reported in the United States. Because many milder cases are not diagnosed or reported, the actual number of infections may be thity or more times greater. Salmonellosis is more common in the summer than winter.

Children are the most likely to get salmonellosis. Young children, the elderly, and the immunocompromised are the most likely to have severe infections. It is estimated that approximately 600 persons die each year with acute salmonellosis.

WHAT ELSE CAN BE DONE TO PREVENT SALMONELLOSIS?

It is important for the public health department to know about cases of salmonellosis. It is important for clinical laboratories to send isolates of *Salmonella* to the City, County, or State Public Health Laboratories so the specific type can be determined and compared with other *Salmonella* in the community. If many cases occur at the same time, it may mean that a restaurant, food or water supply has a problem which needs correction by the public health department.

Some prevention steps occur everyday without you thinking about it. Pasteurization of milk and treating municipal water supplies are highly effective prevention measures that have been in place for many years. In the 1970s, small pet turtles were a common source of salmonellosis in the United States, and in 1975, the sale of small turtles was halted in this country. Improvements in farm animal hygiene, in slaughter plant practices, and in vegetable and fruit harvesting and packing operations may help prevent salmonellosis caused by contaminated foods. Better education of food industry workers in basic food safety and restaurant inspection procedures, may prevent cross-contamination and other food handling errors that can lead to outbreaks. Wider use of pasteurized egg in restaurants, hospitals, and nursing homes is an important prevention measure. In the future, irradiation or other treatments may greatly reduce contamination of raw meat.

WHAT IS THE GOVERNMENT DOING ABOUT SALMONELLOSIS?

The Centers for Disease Control and Prevention (CDC) monitors the frequency of *Salmonella* infections in the country and assists the local and State Health Departments to investigate outbreaks and devise control measures. CDC also conducts research to better identify specific types of *Salmonella*. The Food and Drug Administration inspects imported foods, milk pasteurization plants, promotes better food preparation techniques in restaurants and food processing plants, and regulates the sale of turtles. The FDA also regulates the use of specific antibiotics as growth promotants in food animals. The U.S. Department of Agriculture monitors the health of food animals, inspects egg pasteurization plants, and is responsible for the quality of slaughtered and processed meat. The U.S. Environmental Protection Agency regulates and monitors the safety of our drinking water supplies.

HOW CAN I LEARN MORE ABOUT THIS AND OTHER PUBLIC HEALTH PROBLEMS?

You can discuss any medical concerns you may have with your doctor or other heath care provider. Your local City or County Health Department can provide more information about this and other public health problems that are occurring in your area. General information about the public health of the nation is published every week in the "Morbidity and Mortality Weekly Report", by the CDC in Atlanta, GA. Epidemiologists in your local and State Health Departments are tracking a number of important public health

Appendix

problems, investigating special problems that arise, and helping to prevent them from occurring in the first place, or from spreading if they do occur.

WHAT CAN I DO TO PREVENT SALMONELLOSIS?

- Cook poultry, ground beef, and eggs thoroughly before eating. Do not eat or drink foods containing raw eggs, or raw unpasteurized milk.

- If you are served undercooked meat, poultry or eggs in a restaurant, don't hesitate to send it back to the kitchen for further cooking.

- Wash hands, kitchen work surfaces, and utensils with soap and water immediately after they have been in contact with raw meat or poultry.

- Be particularly careful with foods prepared for infants, the elderly, and the immunocompromised.

- Wash hands with soap after handling reptiles or birds, or after contact with pet feces.

- Avoid direct or even indirect contact between reptiles (turtles, iguanas, other lizards, snakes) and infants or immunocompromised persons.

- Don't work with raw poultry or meat, and an infant (e.g., feed, change diaper) at the same time.

- Mother's milk is the safest food for young infants. Breast-feeding prevents salmonellosis and many other health problems.

Anaerobic—Capable of living and growing without oxygen.

Analgesic—A drug that reduces or eliminates pain.

Antibiotic—A drug that is used to stop the growth of bacteria.

Antibiotic resistance—The ability of a microorganism to destroy or remain unaffected by a drug used against it.

Antibodies—Proteins produced by the immune system to attack and destroy foreign materials that enter the body.

Aquaculture—The farming of plants and animals that live in water, such as fish, shellfish, and algae.

Asymptomatic—Showing no symptoms of disease.

Attachment—The process by which a bacterium connects to a cell it is trying to infect.

Bacillus—A rod-shaped bacterium.

Bacterium (plural is *bacteria*)—A microorganism that can live in nature or infect a host.

Chemical—A substance that is made of molecules and is produced by or used in a reaction.

Colostrum—The thin yellowish fluid secreted by the mammary glands at the time of birth that is rich in antibodies and minerals.

Cytokine—A type of protein released by the body as part of the immune response.

Defecate—To have a bowel movement.

Deoxyribonucleic acid (**DNA**)—A highly complex chemical inside living cells that carries the organism's genetic information.

Encode—To specify the genetic code for a molecule; for example, a protein molecule.

Enteric fever—An infection caused by the bacterium *Salmonella typhosa* that causes fever, weakness, and inflammation and ulceration of the intestines.

Epithelial cell—A specific type of cell that covers most of the internal organs and many of the internal and external surfaces of the body.

Evisceration—A step in the process of animal slaughter during which the contents of the chest and belly cavities of the animal are removed.

Glossary

Fatality rate—The number of deaths that occur in a population from a particular cause over a given amount of time, often expressed as number of deaths per 1,000 of the population per year.

Fecal-oral route—A method of disease transmission whereby the material from the stool of a person with an infectious disease ends up coming into contact with another person's mouth, often by way of water that has been improperly treated.

Filter feeder—An animal that eats by straining particles of food from the water in which it lives.

Fomite—A nonliving object that is capable of spreading pathogens.

Food-borne illness—Sickness that results from consuming contaminated foods or beverages.

Gastroenteritis—Inflammation of the stomach and intestines that is usually accompanied by upset stomach and diarrhea.

Gene—A sequence of DNA present in the cells of all living organisms that determines the particular physical and functional characteristics of the organism.

Gram-negative—Refers to a category of bacteria that, because of their unique structure, do not hold a purple stain used in a particular laboratory test. These cells have a type of bacterial cell wall that is high in lipids and low in peptidoglycan content.

Host—The human, plant, or animal on which or in which another organism lives.

Immune response—Any of several highly specialized reactions the body launches to protect itself against foreign substances.

Immunocompromised—Incapable of developing a normal immune response, usually as a result of disease, malnutrition, or drugs that suppress the immune system.

Incubation period—The period of time between a person's exposure to a disease-causing agent and the first signs of disease.

Infection—A disease that results from the presence and activity of micro-organisms on or in the body.

Isolate—A pathogen or mixture of pathogens taken from a particular source.

Lysosome—A sack-like structure found inside most cells. Lysosomes contain chemicals that are designed to kill bacteria and dissolve materials that enter the cell.

Macrophage—A large phagocytic cell (a cell that engulfs debris and foreign matter).

Malaise—A vague feeling of bodily discomfort and fatigue.

Microvilli (singular is *microvillus*)—Small, fingerlike structures that project from the surface of certain types of cells, such as those that line the small intestine.

Mortality rate—See **Fatality rate**.

Mutation—A change in the genetic material of an organism that results in the creation of a new characteristic or trait or the loss of an existing characteristic or trait.

Niche—The particular combination of nutrition, shelter, and other factors an organism needs to live and grow.

Normal flora—The microorganisms that normally live on and in the body without causing disease.

Nosocomial transmission—The spread of an infectious disease between people in a hospital.

Opportunistic pathogen—A microorganism that can cause disease in people whose immune systems are compromised.

Organism—An individual living thing.

Parasite—An organism that grows, feeds, and is sheltered on or in a different organism and that causes harm to that organism.

Pasteurize—To heat a beverage or food during production in order to kill microorganisms that could cause disease or spoilage.

Pathogen—A microscopic organism that is able to cause a disease.

Pathogenesis—The process by which a pathogen causes disease.

Plasmid—A circular, double-stranded unit of DNA that replicates within a cell independently of the chromosomal DNA. Plasmids are most often found in bacteria and are used in recombinant DNA research to transfer genes between cells.

Glossary

Pili—A hair-like structure, especially on the surface of a cell or microorganism, used for movement, conjugation, and pathogenesis.

Pyogenic—Causing the production of pus.

Pyrogenic—Producing a fever.

Reservoir—An organism or a population that directly or indirectly transmits a pathogen while being virtually immune to its effects.

Ribonucleic acid (RNA)—A constituent of all living cells and many viruses, usually a single-stranded chain of alternating phosphate and ribose units with the bases of adenine, guanine, cytosine, and uracil.

Ribosome—A minute particle composed of RNA and protein that is found in the cytoplasm of living cells.

RNA—See *Ribonucleic acid.*

Salmonellosis—A type of food poisoning that often occurs when a person consumes a food or beverage that contains *Salmonella* bacteria.

Self-limiting—Term used to describe a disease that runs its course without treatment.

Sepsis—A toxic condition resulting from the presence of bacteria or their products in the bloodstream.

Sequencing—Process by which the arrangement of DNA in a gene is identified.

Serotype—A group of closely related microorganisms that share certain structural features.

Shed—Release infectious microorganisms from the body into the environment, as through coughing, sneezing, or excretion.

Spontaneous mutation—A naturally occurring change in the genetic material of an organism that results in the creation of a characteristic or trait that the organism previously lacked.

Systemic—Relating to or affecting the entire body.

Toxin—A poison.

Transformation—The alteration of a bacterial cell caused by the transfer of genetic material from another bacterial cell, especially one capable of causing disease.

Vaccine—A drug made from a weakened or killed pathogen that stimulates a person's immune system to produce antibodies to protect the body against the pathogen.

Vacuole—A small cavity in the cytoplasm of a cell, bound by a single membrane, often containing water, food, or metabolic waste.

Vagus nerve—Either of the cranial nerves that control such functions as speech, swallowing, and the vomit reflex.

Virulence—The ability of a pathogen to cause disease.

Virus—A very small microorganism that can only live inside host cells, and often causes disease. Viruses are not considered living things.

Zoonosis (plural is *zoonoses*)—A disease that can be transmitted from animals to humans.

Bibliography

Alpuche-Aranda, C. M., E. P. Berthiaume, B. Mock, J. A. Swanson, and S. I. Miller. "Spacious Phagosome Formation Within Mouse Macrophages Correlates With *Salmonella* Serotype, Pathogenicity, and Host Susceptibility." *Infection and Immunity* 63 (1995): 4456–4462.

"Antibiotic Characterizations." Available online at *http://www.gpnotebook.co.uk*.

"Antimicrobial Resistance." Centers for Disease Control and Prevention. Available online at *http://www.cdc.gov/drugresistance/index.htm*.

Ask a Scientist. "Bacteria and Stomach Acid." Available online at *http://www.newton.dep.anl.gov/askasci/mole00.mole00179.htm*.

"Bad Taste: *Salmonella* Attack." Available online at *http://www.channel4.com/science/microsites.B/bodystory/bad_salmon.htm*.

Baumler, A. J., R. M. Tsolis, F. A. Bowe, J. G. Kusters, S. Hoffmann, and F. Heffron. "The pef Fimbrial Operon of *Salmonella typhimurium* Mediates Adhesion to Murine Small Intestine and Is Necessary for Fluid Accumulation in the Infant Mouse." *Infection and Immunity* 64 1996: 61–68.

Bej, A. K., M. H. Mahbubani, M. J. Boyce, and R. M. Atlas. "Detection of *Salmonella* spp. in Oysters by PCR." *Applied and Environmental Microbiology* 60 (1) (1994): 368–373.

Centers for Disease Control and Prevention. Available online at *http://www.cdc.gov*.

———. *Morbidity and Mortality Weekly Report*. Available online at *http://www.cdc.gov/mmwr/*.

Chen, L. M., K. Kaniga, and J. E. Galán. "*Salmonella* Spp. Are Cytotoxic for Cultured Macrophages" *Molecular Microbiology* 21 (1996): 1101–1115.

Corcoran, J. W. "Molecular Biology of Sensitivity and Resistance to Antimicrobial Agents." *The Biologic and Clinical Basis of Infectious Disease*. Philadelphia: W. B. Saunders Company, 1985, pp. 756–780.

"Discovery of Antibiotics." Available online at *http://www.molbio.princeton.edu/courses/mb427/2001/projects/02/antibiotics.htm*.

Division of Bacterial and Mycotic Diseases: Food-borne and Diarrheal Diseases Branch. Centers for Disease Control and Prevention. Available online at *http://www.cdc.gov/ncidod/dbmd/food-borne/index.htm*.

Fedorka-Cray, P. J., D. A. Dargatz, L. A. Thomas, and J. T. Gray. "Survey of *Salmonella* Serotypes in Feedlot Cattle." *Journal of Food Protection* 61(5) (1998): 525–530.

Gordon, J. S. "The Passion of Typhoid Mary, Mary Mallon Could Do One Thing Very Well, and All She Wanted Was to Be Left to It." *American Heritage* 45(3) (1994): 118–120.

Heinitz, M. L., D. R. Ruble, D. E. Wagner, and S. R. Tatini. "Incidence of *Salmonella* in Fish and Seafood." *Journal of Food Protection* 63(5) (2000): 579–592.

Howard Hughes Medical Institute. "*Salmonella* Biointeractive Animation Console." Available online at *http://www.hhmi.org/biointeractive/animations/salmonella/sal_print.htm.*

"How Bacteria Become Resistant." Available online at *http://www.abc.net.au/science/slab/antibiotics/resistance.htm.*

"How Do Bacteria Become Resistant to Antibiotics?" Available online at *http://health.howstuffworks.com/question561.htm.*

Hueck, C. J. "Type III Protein Secretion Systems in Bacterial Pathogens of Animals and Plants" *Microbiology and Molecular Biology Reviews* 62(2) (1998): 379–433.

Infectious Disease Information. National Center for Infectious Disease. Centers for Disease Control and Prevention. Available online at *http://www.cdc.gov/ncidod/diseases/submenus/.htm.*

Kiessling, C. R., J. H. Cutting, M. Loftis, W. M. Kiessling, A. R. Datta, and J. N. Sofos. "Antimicrobial Resistance of Food-Related *Salmonella* Isolates, 1999–2000." *Journal of Food Protection* 5(4) (2002): 603–608.

Libby, S. J., T. A, Halsey, C. Altier, J. Potter, C. L. Gyles. "*Salmonella*." *Pathogenesis of Bacterial Infections in Animals*, 3rd ed. Oxford, England: Blackwell Publishing, 2004.

Molla, B., D. Alemayehu, and W. Salah. "Sources and Distribution of *Salmonella* Serotypes Isolated From Food Animals, Slaughterhouse Personnel and Retail Meat Products in Ethiopia: 1997–2002." *Ethiopian Journal of Health* 17(1) (2003): 63–70.

Moore, R. "Outbreak of Multidrug-Resistant *Salmonella* Newport." *Journal of the American Medical Association* 288 (2002): 951–953.

Morello, J. A., and E. E. Baker. "Interaction of *Salmonella* With Phagocytes *in vitro*." *The Journal of Infectious Diseases* 115 (1965): 131–141.

Patterson, S., and R. E. Isaacson. "Genetics and Pathogenesis of *Salmonella*." *Microbial Food Safety in Animal Agriculture: Current Topics*. Iowa City: Iowa State Press, 2003.

Bibliography

PHLIS: Public Health Laboratory Information System. Centers for Disease Control and Prevention. Available online at *http://www.cdc.gov/ncidod/dbmd/phlisdata/default.htm*.

"*Salmonella* as a Bioware Agent?" Available online at *http://www.bt.cdc.gov/agent/agentlist.asp*.

"Serotyping of *Salmonella* Isolates." *Salmonella* Annual Summary 2002. Available online at *http://www.cdc.gov/ncidod/dbmd/phlisdata/salmtab/2002/SalmonellaIntroduction2002.pdf*.

Singer, R. "Antimicrobial Resistance in Food-borne Organisms." *Microbial Food Safety in Animal Agriculture: Current Topics.* Iowa City: Iowa State Press, 2003.

Slauch, J., R. Taylor, and S. Maloy. "Survival in a Cruel World: How *Vibrio cholerae* and *Salmonella* Respond to an Unwilling Host." *Genes and Development* 11(14) (1997): 1761–1774.

Sommers, H. M. "Infectious Diarrhea." *The Biologic and Clinical Basis of Infectious Disease.* Philadelphia: W. B. Saunders Company, 1985, pp. 496–551.

———. "Laboratory Diagnosis of Bacterial Infections." *The Biologic and Clinical Basis of Infectious Disease.* Philadelphia: W. B. Saunders Company, 1985, pp. 119–139.

Torrence, M. E., and R. E. Isaacson. *Microbial Food Safety in Animal Agriculture: Current Topics.* Iowa City: Iowa State Press, 2003.

Tortora, G. J., B. R. Funke, and C. L. Case. *Microbiology: An Introduction,* 7th ed. New York: Benjamin Cummings, 2002.

"Who Discovered *Salmonella*?" Available online at *http://www.whonamedit.com/synd.cfm/402.html*.

Wilson I. G., and J. E. Moore. "Presence of *Salmonella* spp. and *Campylobacter* spp. in Shellfish." *Epidemiology and Infection* 116(2) (1996): 147–153.

Youmans, G. P. "Host-Bacteria interactions: Immunologic Internal Defense Mechanisms." *The Biologic and Clinical Basis of Infectious Disease.* Philadelphia: W. B. Saunders Company, 1985, pp. 25–34.

Bell, C., and A. Kyriakides. *Salmonella: A Practical Approach to the Organism and Its Control in Foods.* Boston: Blackwell Publishers, 2002.

Biology of Salmonella. Dordrecht, Netherlands: Kluwer Academic Publishing, 1993.

"*Escherichia coli* and *Salmonella:* Cellular and Molecular Biology." Washington, D.C.: American Society for Microbiology Press, 1996.

"Evaluation of the *Salmonella* problem." Washington, D.C.: National Academies Press, 1985, pp. 72–103.

Herikstad, H., P. Hayes, M. Mokhtar, M. L. Fracaro, E. J. Threfall, and F. J. Angluo. "Emerging Quinolone-Resistant *Salmonella* in the United States." *Emerging Infectious Diseases* 3 (3) (1997): 371–372.

Hirshmann, K. *Salmonella.* Ann Arbor: Gale, 2003.

Hutwagner, L. C., E. K. Maloney, N. H. Bean, L. Slutsker, and S. M. Martin. "Using Laboratory-Based Surveillance Data for Prevention: An Algorithm for Detecting *Salmonella* Outbreaks." *Emerging Infectious Diseases* 3(3) (1997): 395–400.

Kelterborn, E. *Catalogue of* Salmonella *First Isolations, 1965–1984.* Dordrecht, Netherlands: Kluwer Academic Publishers, 1987.

Libby, S. J., T. A., Halsey, C. Altier, J. Potter, and C. L. Gyles. "*Salmonella.*" *Pathogenesis of Bacterial Infections in Animals*, 3rd ed. Boston: Blackwell Publishing, 2004.

Pascoe, E. *Spreading Menace:* Salmonella *Attack and the Hunger Craving.* Ann Arbor: Gale, 2003.

Report on Salmonella *in Eggs.* Ministry of Agriculture. Lanham, MD: Bernan Associates Publishing, 1993.

Rice, D. H., D. D. Hancock, P. M. Roozen, M. H. Szymanski, B. C. Sheenstra, K. M. Cady, T. E. Besser, and P. A. Chudek. "Household Contamination With *Salmonella enterica.*" *Emerging Infectious Diseases* 9(1) (2003): 120–122.

"Risk Assessments of *Salmonella* in Eggs and Broiler Chickens." Food and Agriculture Organization of the United Nations Publishing (WHO). Geneva, Switzerland. 2nd ed. 2002.

Saeed, A. M., R. Gast, M. E. Potter, and P. G. Wall. Salmonella enterica *Serovar Enteritidis in Humans and Animals: Epidemiology, Pathogenesis, and Control.* Iowa City: Iowa State Press, 1999.

Further Reading

Salmonella: *A Medical Dictionary, Bibliography, and Annotated Research Guide to Internet References.* San Diego: Icon Health Publications, 2004.

Wray, C., and A. Wray. Salmonella *in Domestic Animals.* Cambridge, MA: CABI Publishing, 2001.

Websites

Animal and Plant Health Inspection Services
www.aphis.usda.gov

Centers for Disease Control and Prevention
www.cdc.gov

Emerging Infectious Diseases online journal
www.cdc.gov/ncidod/EID/index.htm

National Center for Infectious Disease
www.cdc.gov/ncidod/diseases/submenus/sub_salmonella.htm

National Institutes of Health
www.nih.gov

PHLIS Surveillance. *Salmonella* annual summaries, 1995–2002
www.cdc.gov/ncidod/dbmd/phlisdata/salmonella.htm

United States Department of Agriculture
www.usda.gov

Index

Index

Picture Credits

About the Author

Danielle Brands is originally from southern California, but moved to Tempe, Arizona, during her sophomore year of high school. After high school, she attended the University of Arizona in Tucson, Arizona, where she started working in a microbiology research laboratory. Brands received her B.S. in 2001 from the University of Arizona in molecular and cellular biology with minors in chemistry, math, and physics. She continued her education at the University of Arizona, receiving an M.S. in pathobiology in 2003. Her Master's project involved testing oysters for the presence of *Salmonella* and *Campylobacter jejuni.*

She currently lives in Tucson, Arizona, with her husband. Brands is currently employed by Ventana Medical Systems, Inc. of Tucson, Arizona, where she is an associate scientist. She is a part of the research and development team that works on cancer detection kits.

About the Founding Editor

The late I. Edward Alcamo was a Distinguished Teaching Professor of Microbiology at the State University of New York at Farmingdale. Alcamo studied biology at Iona College in New York and earned his M.S. and Ph.D. degrees in microbiology at St. John's University, also in New York. He had taught at Farmingdale for over 30 years. In 2000, Alcamo won the Carski Award for Distinguished Teaching in Microbiology, the highest honor for microbiology teachers in the United States. He was a member of the American Society for Microbiology, the National Association of Biology Teachers, and the American Medical Writers Association. Alcamo authored numerous books on the subjects of microbiology, AIDS, and DNA technology as well as the award-winning textbook *Fundamentals of Microbiology,* now in its sixth edition.